T0226435

Headache and Chiari Malformation

Editor

NORIKO SALAMON

NEUROIMAGING CLINICS OF NORTH AMERICA

www.neuroimaging.theclinics.com

Consulting Editor
SURESH K. MUKHERJI

May 2019 • Volume 29 • Number 2

ELSEVIER

1600 John F. Kennedy Boulevard • Suite 1800 • Philadelphia, Pennsylvania, 19103-2899

http://www.neuroimaging.theclinics.com

NEUROIMAGING CLINICS OF NORTH AMERICA Volume 29, Number 2
May 2019 ISSN 1052-5149, ISBN 13: 978-0-323-67782-0

Editor: John Vassallo (j.vassallo@elsevier.com)
Developmental Editor: Casey Potter

Neuroimaging Clinics of North America (ISSN 1052-5149) is published quarterly by Elsevier Inc., 360 Park Avenue South, New York, NY 10010-1710. Months of issue are February, May, August, and November. Business and editorial offices: 1600 John F. Kennedy Blvd., Suite 1800, Philadelphia, PA 19103-2899. Business and editorial offices: 6277 Sea Harbor Drive, Orlando, FL 32887-4800. Periodicals postage paid at New York, NY, and additional mailing offices. Subscription prices are USD 397 per year for US individuals, USD 653 per year for US institutions, USD 100 per year for US students and residents, USD 451 per year for Canadian individuals, USD 832 per year for Canadian institutions, USD 525 per year for international individuals, USD 832 per year for international institutions and USD 260 per year for Canadian and foreign students and residents. To receive student/resident rate, orders must be accompanied by name of affiliated institution, date of term, and the *signature* of program/residency coordinator on institution letterhead. Orders will be billed at individual rate until proof of status is received. Foreign air speed delivery is included in all *Clinics* subscription prices. All prices are subject to change without notice. POSTMASTER: Send address changes to *Neuroimaging Clinics of North America*, Elsevier Health Sciences Division, Subscription **Customer Service, 3251 Riverport Lane, Maryland Heights, MO 63043. Telephone: 1-800-654-2452 (U.S. and Canada); 314-447-8871 (outside U.S. and Canada). Fax: 314-447-8029. E-mail: journalscustomer service-usa@elsevier.com (for print support); journalsonlinesupport-usa@elsevier.com (for online support)**.

Reprints. For copies of 100 or more of articles in this publication, please contact the Commercial Reprints Department, Elsevier Inc., 360 Park Avenue South, New York, NY 10010-1710. Tel.: 212-633-3874; Fax: 212-633-3820; E-mail: reprints@elsevier.com.

Neuroimaging Clinics of North America is covered by *Excerpta Medical/EMBASE,* the RSNA Index of Imaging Literature, *MEDLINE/PubMed (Index Medicus),* MEDLINE/MEDLARS, SciSearch, Research Alert, and Neuroscience Citation Index.

PROGRAM OBJECTIVE

The goal of *Neuroimaging Clinics of North America* is to keep practicing radiologists and radiology residents up to date with current clinical practice in radiology by providing timely articles reviewing the state of the art in patient care.

TARGET AUDIENCE

Practicing radiologists, radiology residents, and other healthcare professionals who utilize neuroimaging findings to provide patient care.

LEARNING OBJECTIVES

Upon completion of this activity, participants will be able to:
1. Review the application of advanced imaging for the diagnosis and treatment of the headache
2. Discuss the clinical evaluation of children with headache
3. Recognize major causes of headaches including sinus disease, Chiari malformation, and aneurysm.

ACCREDITATION

The Elsevier Office of Continuing Medical Education (EOCME) is accredited by the Accreditation Council for Continuing Medical Education (ACCME) to provide continuing medical education for physicians.

The EOCME designates this enduring material for a maximum of 15 *AMA PRA Category 1 Credit*(s)™. Physicians should claim only the credit commensurate with the extent of their participation in the activity.

All other healthcare professionals requesting continuing education credit for this enduring material will be issued a certificate of participation.

DISCLOSURE OF CONFLICTS OF INTEREST

The EOCME assesses conflict of interest with its instructors, faculty, planners, and other individuals who are in a position to control the content of CME activities. All relevant conflicts of interest that are identified are thoroughly vetted by EOCME for fair balance, scientific objectivity, and patient care recommendations. EOCME is committed to providing its learners with CME activities that promote improvements or quality in healthcare and not a specific proprietary business or a commercial interest.

The planning committee, staff, authors and editors listed below have identified no financial relationships or relationships to products or devices they or their spouse/life partner have with commercial interest related to the content of this CME activity:

Abraham F. Bezuidenhout, MD; Rafeeque A. Bhadelia, MD; Sarah Cantrell, MD; Stephen M. Chan, MD; Yu-Ming Chang, MD, PhD; Andrew C. Charles, MD; Yosef G. Chodakiewitz, MD; Nicholas R. Dudeck, BS; Benjamin M. Ellingson, PhD; Judith A. Gadde, DO, MBA; Wende N. Gibbs, MD, MA; Shahram Hadidchi, MD; Carl B. Heilman, MD; Chelsea Hesterman, MD; Mollie Johnston, MD; Alison Kemp; Yasufumi Kijima, MD, PhD; Paul E. Kim, MD; Preetham Kumar, MD; Pradeep Kuttysankaran; O-Ki Kwon, MD, PhD; Alexander Lerner, MD; Chia-Shang Jason Liu, MD, PhD; Marcel M. Maya, MD; Franklin G. Moser, MD, MMM; Suresh K. Mukherji, MD, MBA, FACR; Mark E. Mullins, MD, PhD; Sumir S. Patel, MD, MBA; Tina Young Poussaint, MD, FACR; Noriko Salamon, MD, PhD; Asha Sarma, MD; Wouter I. Schievink, MD; Mark S. Shiroishi, MD, MS; Wesley Surento, MS; John Vassallo; Juan Pablo Villablanca, MD; Brian H. West, MD, MS.

The planning committee, staff, authors and editors listed below have identified financial relationships or relationships to products or devices they or their spouse/life partner have with commercial interest related to the content of this CME activity:

Claudia F.E. Kirsch, MD: is a consultant/advisor for Informa UK Limited.
Jonathan M. Tobis, MD: is a consultant/advisor for W. L. Gore & Associates, Inc.

UNAPPROVED/OFF-LABEL USE DISCLOSURE

The EOCME requires CME faculty to disclose to the participants:
1. When products or procedures being discussed are off-label, unlabelled, experimental, and/or investigational (not US Food and Drug Administration [FDA] approved); and
2. Any limitations on the information presented, such as data that are preliminary or that represent ongoing research, interim analyses, and/or unsupported opinions. Faculty may discuss information about pharmaceutical agents that is outside of FDA-approved labelling. This information is intended solely for CME and is not intended to promote off-label use of these medications. If you have any questions, contact the medical affairs department of the manufacturer for the most recent prescribing information.

TO ENROLL

To enroll in the *Neuroimaging Clinics of North America* Continuing Medical Education program, call customer service at 1-800-654-2452 or sign up online at http://www.theclinics.com/home/cme. The CME program is available to subscribers for an additional annual fee of USD 244.40.

METHOD OF PARTICIPATION

In order to claim credit, participants must complete the following:

1. Complete enrolment as indicated above.
2. Read the activity.
3. Complete the CME Test and Evaluation. Participants must achieve a score of 70% on the test. All CME Tests and Evaluations must be completed online.

CME INQUIRIES/SPECIAL NEEDS

For all CME inquiries or special needs, please contact elsevierCME@elsevier.com.

NEUROIMAGING CLINICS OF NORTH AMERICA

Contributors

CONSULTING EDITOR

SURESH K. MUKHERJI, MD, MBA, FACR
Professor and Chairman, Walter F. Patenge
Endowed Chair, Department of Radiology,
Michigan State University, Chief Medical
Officer & Director of Health Care Delivery,
Michigan State University Health Team,
East Lansing, Michigan, USA

EDITOR

NORIKO SALAMON, MD, PhD
Professor, Department of Radiology, Section
of Neuroradiology, David Geffen School of
Medicine at University of California,
Los Angeles, Los Angeles, California, USA

AUTHORS

ABRAHAM F. BEZUIDENHOUT, MD
Neuroradiology Fellow, Department of
Radiology, Beth Israel Deaconess Medical
Center, Boston, Massachusetts,
USA

RAFEEQUE A. BHADELIA, MD
Associate Professor, Department of Radiology,
Harvard Medical School, Clinical Director, Staff
Neuroradiologist, Beth Israel Deaconess
Medical Center, Boston, Massachusetts,
USA

SARAH CANTRELL, MD
Baylor Radiologists, CHI St. Lukes, Texas
Medical Center, Houston, Texas,
USA

STEPHEN M. CHAN, MD
Diagnostic Radiology Resident, Cedars-Sinai
Medical Center, Los Angeles, California,
USA

YU-MING CHANG, MD, PhD
Neuroradiology Fellowship Director, Staff
Neuroradiologist, Department of Radiology,
Beth Israel Deaconess Medical Center,
Boston, Massachusetts, USA

ANDREW C. CHARLES, MD
Department of Neurology, David Geffen School
of Medicine, University of California
Los Angeles, Los Angeles, California,
USA

YOSEF G. CHODAKIEWITZ, MD
Diagnostic Radiology Resident, Cedars-Sinai
Medical Center, Los Angeles, California,
USA

NICHOLAS R. DUDECK, BS
UCLA Center for Computer Vision and Imaging
Biomarkers, Department of Radiological
Sciences, David Geffen School of Medicine,
University of California, Los Angeles,
Los Angeles, California, USA

BENJAMIN M. ELLINGSON, PhD
UCLA Center for Computer Vision and Imaging
Biomarkers, Departments of Radiological
Sciences, and Psychiatry and Biobehavioral
Sciences, UCLA Brain Research Institute (BRI),
Associate Professor of Radiology, Biomedical
Physics, Psychiatry, and Bioengineering,
Director, UCLA Brain Tumor Imaging
Laboratory (BTIL), Departments of Radiological
Sciences, and Psychiatry, David Geffen School
of Medicine, University of California, Los
Angeles, Los Angeles, California, USA

JUDITH A. GADDE, DO, MBA
Assistant Professor, Department of Radiology,
Emory University School of Medicine, Atlanta,
Georgia, USA

WENDE N. GIBBS, MD, MA
Division of Neuroradiology, Department of
Radiology, Keck School of Medicine of USC,
University of Southern California, Los Angeles,
California, USA

SHAHRAM HADIDCHI, MD
Division of Neuroradiology, Department of
Radiology, Keck School of Medicine of USC,
University of Southern California, Los Angeles,
California, USA

CARL B. HEILMAN, MD
Chairman, Department of Neurosurgery, Tufts
Medical Center, Boston, Massachusetts,
USA

CHELSEA HESTERMAN, MD
Department of Neurology, David Geffen
School of Medicine, University of California,
Los Angeles, Los Angeles, California,
USA

MOLLIE JOHNSTON, MD
Department of Neurology, David Geffen School
of Medicine, University of California, Los
Angeles, Los Angeles, California, USA

YASUFUMI KIJIMA, MD, PhD
Department of Cardiovascular Medicine,
St. Luke's International Hospital, Tokyo, Japan

PAUL E. KIM, MD
Division of Neuroradiology, Department of
Radiology, Keck School of Medicine of USC,
University of Southern California, Los Angeles,
California, USA

CLAUDIA F.E. KIRSCH, MD
Division Chief of Neuroimaging Service Line,
Professor of Neuroradiology and
Otolaryngology, Department of Radiology,
Northwell Health, Donald and Barbara Zucker
School of Medicine at Hofstra/Northwell,
North Shore University Hospital, Manhasset,
New York, USA

PREETHAM KUMAR, MD
Cardiology, University of California,
Los Angeles, Los Angeles, California, USA

O-KI KWON, MD, PhD
Department of Neurosurgery, Seoul National
University Bundang Hospital, Bundanggu,
Seongnamsi, Gyeonggido, South Korea

ALEXANDER LERNER, MD
Division of Neuroradiology, Department of
Radiology, Keck School of Medicine of USC,
University of Southern California, Los Angeles,
California, USA

CHIA-SHANG JASON LIU, MD, PhD
Division of Neuroradiology, Department of
Radiology, Keck School of Medicine of USC,
University of Southern California, Los Angeles,
California, USA

MARCEL M. MAYA, MD
Co-chair, Department of Imaging,
Cedars-Sinai Medical Center, Los Angeles,
California, USA

FRANKLIN G. MOSER, MD, MMM
Professor of Imaging, Vice Chair of Radiology
Research, Cedars-Sinai Medical Center,
Los Angeles, California, USA

MARK E. MULLINS, MD, PhD
Professor, Department of Radiology, Emory
University School of Medicine, Atlanta,
Georgia, USA

SUMIR S. PATEL, MD, MBA
Assistant Professor, Department of Radiology,
Emory University School of Medicine, Atlanta,
Georgia, USA

TINA YOUNG POUSSAINT, MD, FACR
Professor, Department of Radiology, Harvard
Medical School, Attending Neuroradiologist,
Boston Children's Hospital, Boston,
Massachusetts, USA

ASHA SARMA, MD
Assistant Professor of Radiology
and Radiological Sciences, Department
of Radiology, Vanderbilt University
Medical Center, Monroe Carell Jr. Children's
Hospital, Nashville, Tennessee, USA

WOUTER I. SCHIEVINK, MD
Neurosurgery Professor and Director of
Microvascular Neurosurgery, Cedars-Sinai
Medical Center, Advanced Health Sciences
Pavilion, Los Angeles, California, USA

MARK S. SHIROISHI, MD, MS
Assistant Professor, Division of
Neuroradiology, Department of Radiology,
Visiting Scholar, USC Imaging Genetics
Center, Mark and Mary Stevens Neuroimaging
and Informatics Institute, Keck School of
Medicine of USC, University of Southern
California, Los Angeles, California, USA

WESLEY SURENTO, MS
Division of Neuroradiology, Department of
Radiology, Keck School of Medicine of USC,
University of Southern California, Los Angeles,
California, USA

JONATHAN M. TOBIS, MD
Professor of Medicine, Cardiology, University
of California, Los Angeles, Los Angeles,
California, USA

JUAN PABLO VILLABLANCA, MD
Department of Radiological Sciences, David
Geffen School of Medicine, University of
California, Los Angeles, Los Angeles,
California, USA

BRIAN H. WEST, MD, MS
Cardiology, University of California,
Los Angeles, Los Angeles, California,
USA

Contents

One of the most common reasons that a patient seeks out a health care provider for a neuroscience-related issue is headache. Not all patients can, or probably should, be imaged with headache. We must use an approach that attends to scientific evidence, accepted guidelines, and available resources. This approach should focus on quality, safety, appropriateness, and utilization. This article reviews and discusses the consideration of imaging adult patients with headache.

Review of the clinical presentation, imaging findings, and management of headache secondary to intracranial hypotension.

Headaches and sinus disease are common reasons to seek medical care, with marked worldwide prevalence and large socioeconomic burdens. Headaches caused by sinus diseases are rare; many "rhinogenic headaches" are actually migraines. The similar symptoms may result from autonomic dysfunction and trigeminovascular pathways. Using the mnemonic ACHE, this article presents key Anatomy, Clinical cases, How to image, Essential clinical and radiographic features that help the radiologist, otolaryngologist, and neurologist evaluate sinus disease and headaches.

 Video content accompanies this article at http://www.neuroimaging.theclinics.com.

Headache is a common symptom in patients with Chiari I malformation (CMI), characterized by 5 mm or greater cerebellar tonsillar herniation below foramen magnum. Radiologists should be aware of the different types of headaches reported by CMI patients and which headache patterns are distinctive features of the diagnosis. A methodical imaging strategy is required to fully assess a CMI patient to exclude secondary causes of tonsillar herniation such as intracranial hypotension or associated conditions such as syrinx. Both anatomic and physiologic imaging can help determine if headaches are CMI associated, and assist clinicians in therapeutic decision making.

Headache may be the most common presenting symptom of unruptured intracranial aneurysms. Unruptured intracranial aneurysm can be found in the work-up for headache but direct causality is not clear. Most of the headaches have been thought to be incidental symptoms of unruptured intracranial aneurysms. If high-risk patients with symptoms such as headache could be selected it would help in diagnosing unruptured intracranial aneurysms. Many aspects of unruptured intracranial aneurysm–associated headaches are unclear, including the mechanism, discriminating characteristics, and localization. This article reviews basic knowledge on cerebral aneurysm and headache, and describes the possible mechanism and characteristics of aneurysm-associated headaches.

Observational studies have identified a relationship between patent foramen ovale (PFO) and migraine headache. In people who have migraine with aura, 40% to 60% have a PFO, compared with 20% to 30% in the general adult population. It is hypothesized that migraine, especially migraine with aura, may be triggered by hypoxemia or vasoactive chemicals (eg, serotonin), which are ordinarily metabolized during passage through the lungs. Although PFO closure is currently not a FDA–approved therapy for migraines, randomized trials suggest that this intervention may benefit a subgroup of migraineurs.

Pediatric headache is a common problem, with various underlying causes. Appropriate patient selection for neuroimaging is necessary to optimize the clinical evaluation. This review aims to provide a focused discussion of the clinical evaluation of children with headache, including published guidelines pertaining to neuroimaging, technical considerations for neuroimaging, and tailoring of examinations for specific clinical entities known to cause pediatric headache.

Headaches are exceedingly common, but most individuals who seek medical attention with headache will not have a serious underlying etiology such as a brain tumor. Brain tumors are uncommon; however, many patients with brain tumors do suffer from headaches. Generally these headaches are accompanied by other neurologic signs and symptoms. A careful clinical assessment for red flags should be undertaken when considering further work-up with neuroimaging to exclude a serious underlying condition.

The use of advanced imaging in routine diagnostic practice appears to provide only limited value in patients with migraine who have not experienced recent changes in headache characteristics or symptoms. However, advanced imaging may have potential for studying the biological manifestations and pathophysiology of migraine headaches. Migraine with aura appears to have characteristic spatiotemporal changes in structural anatomy, function, hemodynamics, metabolism, and biochemistry, whereas migraine without aura produces more subtle and complex changes. Large, controlled, multicenter imaging-based observational trials are needed to confirm the anecdotal evidence in the literature and test the scientific hypotheses thought to underscore migraine pathophysiology.

Foreword
Headache and Chiari Malformation

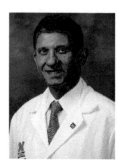

Suresh K. Mukherji, MD, MBA, FACR
Consulting Editor

Headaches are one of the most challenging medical topics that affects our health care system at so many levels. There are innumerable causes of headache that are due to a variety of factors, and one of the major challenges is to identify which patients have organic causes and when it is appropriate to image.

This issue focuses on this difficult topic, and I am extremely grateful to Dr Noriko Salamon for agreeing to guest-edit this important issue of *Neuroimaging Clinics*. She has assembled an "all-star" group of authors who have done a wonderful job of composing beautifully written and illustrated articles. The issue covers a variety of important topics with a specific article dedicated to appropriate imaging and the socioeconomic impact on our health care system.

I want to personally thank Dr Salamon and all the authors for their impressive contributions. This unique issue will be helpful to all health care specialists who are involved in the care of patients with headaches. This important contribution will help improve our understanding of this difficult topic and reduce our "headaches" about "headache"!

Suresh K. Mukherji, MD, MBA, FACR
Department of Radiology
Michigan State University
Michigan State University Health Team
846 Service Road
East Lansing, MI 48824, USA

E-mail address:
mukherji@rad.msu.edu

https://doi.org/10.1016/j.nic.2019.02.002
1052-5149/19/© 2019 Published by Elsevier Inc.

neuroimaging.theclinics.com

Preface

State-of-the-Art Imaging and Current Status of Headaches

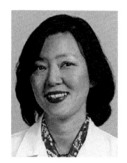

Noriko Salamon, MD, PhD
Editor

Headache is a very common problem and is affected by a spectrum of diseases. Neuroimaging has been playing an important role in making a diagnosis and in the treatment planning of patients.

In this issue, I attempt to cover the usual and multiple causes of headaches that anyone can encounter routinely in practice. Headache is the tip of the iceberg of many different clinical conditions, and the treatment decision should be made quickly based on the imaging findings.

First, I would like to express my gratitude to the consulting editor, Dr Suresh Mukherji, for giving me an opportunity to be a guest editor for this issue of *Neuroimaging Clinics*.

All the authors of this issue are experts in each of their topics, and the readers receive a comprehensive review and learn novel aspects of headaches and imaging. The first article includes an overview of the current practice in patients with headaches, followed by detailed diagnosis and treatment of the intracranial hypotension/cerebrospinal fluid leak. Then, we discuss major causes of headaches, including sinus disease, Chiari malformation, and aneurysm. Patent foramen ovale (PFO) can be related to stroke or migraine, and treatment

of PFO can be useful in the treatment of headaches. Pediatric headaches need to be approached differently. Brain tumor is one of the most serious causes of headaches. And we cover the application of advanced imaging for the diagnosis and treatment of headaches.

I would like to thank all of the expert authors of this issue for accepting my invitation and for their excellent contributions.

Finally, I would like to sincerely thank the series editor, John Vassallo, and the developmental editor, Casey Potter, at Elsevier, for their kind, tireless guidance and support during the entire course of preparation.

Noriko Salamon, MD, PhD
Department of Radiology
Section of Neuroradiology
David Geffen School of Medicine
University of California, Los Angeles
757 Westwood Plaza, Suite 1621D
Los Angeles, CA 90095, USA

E-mail address:
nsalamon@mednet.ucla.edu

Neuroimag Clin N Am 29 (2019) xvii
https://doi.org/10.1016/j.nic.2019.02.001
1052-5149/19/© 2019 Published by Elsevier Inc.

Neuroimaging of Adults with Headache
Appropriateness, Utilization, and an Economical Overview

Judith A. Gadde, DO, MBA[a],*, Sarah Cantrell, MD[b],
Sumir S. Patel, MD, MBA[a], Mark E. Mullins, MD, PhD[a]

KEYWORDS

- Adult • Appropriateness • Headache • Imaging • Indication • Quality • Safety • Socioeconomics

KEY POINTS

- Attention to quality, safety, utilization, and appropriateness will benefit both patients presenting with headache, as well as the health care system.
- The cost of headache to the individual patient can be large, as can the cost to society.
- Becoming familiar with the workup and treatment of headaches will typically make one a better neuroradiologist.

BACKGROUND AND IMPORTANCE

An approach to thinking about the workup of patients for referral to the Radiology department is nicely phrased in the abstract of an article from Lester and Liu: "When deciding to perform imaging for headache, it is important to consider many factors including the pretest probability, prevalence of diseases, sensitivity of imaging, and implications of treatment."[1] It is hoped that the reader will agree that this approach is not unique to the workup of patients with headache.

This article is meant to complement the others in this issue of *Neuroimaging Clinics of North America* and is organized with attention to quality, safety, utilization, and appropriateness, including socioeconomics. This work is not meant to be all-inclusive because that would likely require the length of 1 or more books. To help with focus, this article attends to adults; as well, the emphasis of this work is on nontraumatic presentations. Health care resources are typically limited; appropriate utilization of resources is paramount to the practice of medicine.

Frequency

Although many of us view headache as a ubiquitous aspect of life, studies demonstrate an estimated overall lifetime prevalence of headache (any kind) between 0.2% and 60%.[2] Headaches are most common between the ages of 25 and 55 years.[2] Hainer and Matheson estimated in 2013 that half of the world's adult population suffered from a "headache disorder."[3]

According to the World Health Organization, headache disorders are estimated to have affected half of all people within the last year.[4] Two to four percent of visits to Emergency Departments (EDs) are due to nontraumatic headaches,

J.A. Gadde and S. Cantrell are co-first authors.
There are no commercial or financial conflicts of interest or any funding sources for any authors.
[a] Department of Radiology, Emory University School of Medicine, 1364 Clifton Road NE, BG 20, Atlanta, GA 30322, USA; [b] Baylor Radiologists, CHI St Lukes, Texas Medical Center, 6720 Bertner Avenue, MC 2-270, Houston, Texas 77030, USA
* Corresponding author.
E-mail address: jagadde@emory.edu

Neuroimag Clin N Am 29 (2019) 203–211
https://doi.org/10.1016/j.nic.2019.01.001

with more than 800,000 annual ED visits due to migraine.[5–7] Although ED use for the workup and treatment of uncomplicated headache is likely suboptimal for multiple reasons (including but not limited to especially limited resources, long wait times, and characteristic lack of care continuity), approximately 5 million people per year seek headache treatment in the ED.[6]

Epidemiology

Although different types of headaches have typically varying age and gender distribution, headache disorders overall show no clear distinction between gender, race, age, geography, and income.[4,8] Furthermore, headache disorders, including migraine and medication-overuse headache, result in the third highest worldwide cause of disability when measured in years of life with disability.[9,10] Even though there is such a high prevalence of headache, it is estimated that only 50% of migraine sufferers in the United States sought professional (health) care for this issue in the last year.[4]

Appropriateness

In the mid-1980s, the RAND/UCLA Appropriateness Method defined an appropriate procedure as one in which "the expected health benefit exceeds the expected negative consequences by a sufficiently wide margin that the procedure is worth doing, exclusive of cost."[11] The ACR (American College of Radiology) Appropriateness Criteria (ACR AC), which will also be discussed later, assists in determining when and what kind of neuroimaging is appropriate for use in patients presenting with headaches.[2]

Utilization

Imaging services and their costs grew at almost twice the rate of our health care technologies during the early 2000s.[12] Overutilization of imaging services may be defined as when imaging procedures are performed despite the unlikeliness to improve patient outcome. As alluded earlier, resources are, almost by their very nature, limited and we must be good stewards of these. The typical radiology modalities used to evaluate patients with headache are computed tomography (CT) and MR imaging.

Quality

Quality assurance is the act of measuring compliance against standards. Quality improvement is the continuous act of increasing quality efforts. Quality assurance can be performed without quality improvement, but not vice versa. This is the era for the service-focused practice of radiology. Providing excellent quality and service is our goal. Constant attention to quality is necessary and assuming (but not confirming) quality work may be folly. Evaluation of patients with headache is not unique in this regard, but a focus on quality should not be overlooked nonetheless.

Safety

More than 15 years after the release of the Institute of Medicine's report, "To Err is Human: Building a Safer Health System," patient safety remains at the forefront of the radiologists' minds.[13] Apropos of imaging of patients with headache, attention to this in our department includes but is not limited to CT with ionizing radiation exposure, MR imaging compatibility, use of contrast material, imaging of pregnant patients, minimizing patient radiation dose, and so on. Related topics include (but are not limited to) ALARA (As Low As Reasonably Allowable),[14] Image Gently,[15] and Image Wisely.[15] As with the earlier mention of quality, a focus on safety when approaching potentially imaging patients with headache is not unique but, it is thought, remains relevant and important.

SPECTRUM OF HEADACHES IN ADULTS

Classification of headaches into either primary or secondary is essential for proper evaluation and treatment. That being said, the clinical diagnosis of headache is beyond the scope of this article. Herein, the authors mention a few of the salient concepts. An axiom of neuroradiology is that being familiar with relevant workups and treatments outside of the Radiology department typically makes one a better neuroradiologist.

Headache Classification in the Adult

The third edition of the International Classification of Headache Disorders (ICHD), developed by the International Headache Society, is commonly accepted worldwide as an evidence-based guideline for the diagnosis and classification of headache disorders.[15,16] The ICHD-3 classifies headaches into 3 main groups: (1) primary headaches; (2) secondary headaches; and (3) "painful cranial neuropathies," "other facial pains," and other headaches.[15]

Primary headaches are those that are usually benign and include (but are not limited to) migraine with or without aura, tension-type headache, cluster headaches, and less common headache disorders such as cold-stimulus, cough, and exertional headache.[17]

Secondary headaches[18] are those caused by an underlying disease, which includes (but are not limited to) both (usually) benign and sinister causes such as sinusitis and subarachnoid hemorrhage, respectively. Secondary headaches tend to be less common than primary headaches; an article from Ravishankar in 2016 estimated "less than 10%."[19] Secondary headaches are further divided into 7 main groups: traumatic headaches (head and/or neck); cranial or cervical vascular disorders; nonvascular intracranial disorders; substance use or withdrawal; infections; headache or facial pain attributed to disorder of the cranium, neck, eyes, ears, nose, sinuses, teeth, mouth, or other facial or cervical structure; and psychiatric disorder.[15,16] Practically, common causes of secondary headache, which may require prompt treatment, include but are not limited to intracranial hemorrhage, aneurysm, meningitis, venous sinus thrombosis, and idiopathic intracranial hypertension amongst many others. One study by Grant[20] found that approximately 23% of patients with a primary brain tumor presented with a headache as the first symptom. An additional retrospective review found that headache was a symptom in 48% of 111 patients with brain tumor.[21] A commonly stated motivation for imaging patients complaining of headache is that "it could be something *bad*" and, practically speaking, that argument is moving but with limited resources not all patients with headache may be imaged always and routinely, and thus some justice- and medically based approach to utilization seems appropriate. Furthermore, it is not clear that all patients with headache should be imaged given possible ionizing radiation exposure, potential contrast material administration, access issues with MR imaging, etc. even if there are unlimited resources, which obviously are not.

Red Flags in Adult Headache

Although most individuals are eventually diagnosed as having migraine and/or tension-type headaches (examples of primary headaches), eliminating the possibility of treatable and/or dangerous causes of secondary headache is critical.[22] Clinical features that raise concern for secondary headache are commonly called "red flags" and use of some of these, including but not limited to "…paralysis; papilledema; and 'drowsiness, confusion, memory impairment and loss of consciousness,'" has been reported to be statistically significant.[23]

According to Clinch in 2001, "'Red flags' for secondary disorders include sudden onset, onset after 50 years of age, increased frequency or severity, new onset with an underlying medical condition, concomitant systemic illness, focal neurologic signs or symptoms, papilledema and headache subsequent to trauma."[17] In 2013, Hainer and Matheson published that red flags in adult patients with headache include "…focal neurologic signs, papilledema, neck stiffness, an immunocompromised state, sudden onset of the worst headache of the patient's life, personality changes, headache after trauma, and headache that is worse with exercise."[3]

To aid physicians in deciding which patients should proceed to neuroimaging for evaluation of clinically significant lesions causing headache (secondary headache), Dodick (2003) introduced the SNOOP mnemonic for the identification of clinical "red flags," which may help distinguish primary and secondary headache.[24] These criteria were further revised and adapted to the emergency room setting by Nye and Ward to include Systemic Illness (eg, fever, chills, human immunodeficiency virus, history of cancer), Neurologic signs (eg, change in mental status, asymmetric reflexes), Onset (eg, acute, sudden or split second thunderclap headache), Older patients (eg, >50 years with new or progressive headache), Previous headache history (eg, first headache or different headache changing in frequency, severity, or clinical features), headache in children younger than 5 years, and headache worsening under observation.[25] Some investigators also use an additional expression entitled "yellow flags."[26]

ECONOMIC BURDEN OF HEADACHE

The cost of headache to the individual patient may be large; the cost to society is also remarkable. Headaches are estimated to result in health care expenses of more than $1 billion annually in the United States. It is estimated that 113 million workdays each year are lost due to headache, resulting in about a $13 to 19.6 billion loss to the US economy.[27,28] For chronic migraineurs alone, a 2011 study found that these patients spend $1036 every 3 months on direct headache-related costs, including diagnostic imaging.[29] For perspective, the average cost of a noncontrast head CT is estimated to be between $682 and $1390.[30] In addition, the average brain MR imaging is estimated to be between $1000 and $5000.[30] **Table 1** includes published price ranges for both of these examinations. An approach to cost-effectiveness in this workup[31] is clearly indicated.

Although there have been increasing efforts in consumer price transparency for health care costs, including imaging, there remains a broad range of "average" costs. As imaging

Table 1
Price ranges for common imaging examinations in the evaluation of headache (healthcarebluebook.com)[34]

	Low (USD, $)	High (USD, $)
Radiograph—Face	28	675
Radiograph—paranasal sinuses	37	912
CT head without contrast	219	1983
CT head without and with contrast	248	3014
CT angiography of the head (with contrast)	630	3219
MR imaging brain without contrast	468	3397
MR imaging brain without and with contrast	468	5354
MR angiography of the head (without contrast)	468	3269

From CAREOperative. Find Your Fair Price. 2018. Available at: https://www.healthcarebluebook.com/ui/consumerfront. Accessed May 24, 2018.

examinations such as these are usually requested by nonradiologists, a suboptimal grasp on the cost of these examinations may contribute to the economic burden imposed on headache sufferers.

Unfortunately, this ignorance of imaging cost does not seem to be restricted to nonradiology trainees. A 2014 online survey of more than 1000 US radiology trainees demonstrated that almost 50% of respondents incorrectly estimated the cost of every imaging examination tested.[32] Almost 90% of study respondents desired more dedicated education regarding imaging costs.[32] Trainees with an advanced degree in health policy or economics and trainees who received dedicated education in these areas did not perform better than those trainees without the advanced degree or dedicated education.[32]

Another survey of almost 400 trainees at a large academic institution demonstrated similar findings with more than 75% of respondents incorrectly estimating the cost of every imaging examination.[33] More than 75% of study respondents also desired that cost data be incorporated into clinical decision support.[33]

As mentioned briefly earlier, **Table 1** includes published low and high price estimates for common imaging examinations used in the evaluation of headache, as found on healthcarebluebook.com.[34] These price estimates can be found by searching for examination type based on zip code.[34]

Economics of Imaging Headache in the Emergency Department and/or the Primary Cary Setting

The evaluation of both primary and secondary headache may be performed not only in the nonacute/nonemergent but also in the emergent setting. It should be noted that in the absence of an abnormal neurologic examination, headache alone has a lower likelihood of resulting in a causative lesion on imaging[35–37]; this is akin to the subsection of migraine headache mentioned earlier. In classic migraine and tension-type headaches, neuroimaging is considered by some investigators to be unnecessary due to the remarkably decreased expected rate of pathology that is usually identified by imaging in these scenarios.[38] Overall, there is a very low reported rate of identifiable intracranial pathology in patients presenting with headache who receive neuroimaging, with individual pathologic prevalence of subdural hematoma, brain tumors, hydrocephalus, arteriovenous malformations, and aneurysm of less than 1%.[39]

Evaluation of Headache in the Emergency Department

Evaluation of headache in the ED typically differs from evaluation in the clinic due to the emphasis on excluding immediately life-threatening causes, the need for efficient management in the ED,[17] and the potential for lack of clinical follow-up by the patient, either in the ED or in the clinic.[40] The consequent sense of urgency and need to initiate potentially life-saving treatment make CT a popular choice of initial test due to its availability, rapid acquisition, and the oftentimes high sensitivity of CT in the evaluation of acutely life-threatening causes. Chillingly, amongst the most common misdiagnosed neurologic complaints in the ED is patients who subsequently follow-up with neurologists for headache.[40]

Challenges related to the clinical setting (ED vs clinic) include, but are not limited to, patient anxiety and desire for imaging as well as fear of litigation; these typically further add to the heterogeneity of imaging workup of headache. An article by Jordan and colleagues[41] noted that "…incremental cost per clinically significant case detected in the ED was $50078." and they concluded that "…emergent CT imaging of nonfocal headache…has limited cost efficacy." It is also of note that some investigators have reported low utilization of neurology consultation in this setting, including Young and colleagues[26] in 2018.

CURRENT (AS OF THE TIME OF THIS WRITING) EVIDENCE-BASED GUIDELINES REGARDING IMAGING OF HEADACHE

American Academy of Neurology Guidelines

Per the report of the Quality Standards Subcommittee of the American Academy of Neurology Evidence-Based Guidelines for Migraine Headache, neuroimaging was not usually warranted in patients with migraine and a normal neurologic examination.[42]

International Headache Society Guidelines

Similarly, the European Headache Federation Consensus on Technical Investigation for Primary Headache Disorders suggested that no imaging is characteristically required in workup of migraine without aura.[43]

National Clinical Guideline Centre

The National Clinical Guideline Centre on behalf of the National Institute for Health and Clinical Excellence states that patients with tension-type headache, migraine, cluster headache, or medication overuse headache should not be imaged for reassurance purposes only.[44]

US Headache Consortium

A 14-member consortium led by the American Academy of Neurology with members from the American Academy of Family Physicians, the American Headache Society, the American College of Emergency Physicians, the American College of Physicians, the American Osteopathic Association, and the National Headache Foundation has produced 5 evidence-based practice guidelines including recommendations for neuroimaging of patients with nonacute headache.[45] These evidence-based guidelines are thus far apparently inadequately used, despite wide availability.[45]

Grade A recommendations are those based on multiple clinical trials with consistent relevant findings.[45] Grade B recommendations are those with some supportive evidence, although the amount of evidence is suboptimal.[45] Grade C recommendations are those without sufficient evidence but developed by a consensus of the US Headache Consortium.[45] No recommendation (Grade C recommendation) is given regarding the comparative sensitivities of CT versus MR imaging.[45]

Some investigators have published that neuroimaging is not warranted in adult patients with migraine, no history of seizures, no change in recent headache patterns, and no focal neurologic sign or symptom (presumably Grade B).[46]

The US Headache Consortium stated that neuroimaging is usually not indicated in patients with a normal neurologic examination in the setting of migraine (also presumably Level B).[45]

American College of Radiology Appropriateness Criteria

It is our understanding that the ACR AC are evidence-based guidelines initially developed in the early 1990s primarily for referring physicians and other providers in an attempt to reduce inappropriate utilization of radiologic services.[47] These guidelines include genres of diagnostic imaging selection, image-guided interventional procedures, and radiotherapy protocols.

There are 16 ACR AC variants currently listed under the clinical condition of headache, including (but not limited to) chronic headaches, sudden onset of headache, and new headaches.[2] A rating system is used to rank each radiologic procedure for each clinical variant. A rating of 1, 2, or 3 is given for procedures that are usually not appropriate for the specific variant.[2] A rating of 4, 5, or 6 suggests the procedure may be appropriate.[2] A rating of 7, 8, or 9 is given for those procedures that are usually appropriate.[2] For example, currently, a CT head with intravenous (IV) contrast is given a rating of 3 for sudden onset of severe headache versus a CT head without IV contrast in this same scenario, which receives a rating of 9.[2]

A comments section is also available for each variant, when clinically relevant. For example, the ACR AC suggest that an MR imaging head without IV contrast may be helpful for sudden onset of severe headache depending on the CT findings.[2]

As well, a relative radiation level is given for each radiologic procedure when pertinent. This level may assist referring physicians in deciding which examination is best for patients, as well as answer questions that patients may have in regard to relative radiation risk or dose. Of note, these provided level assessments are not numeric but more of general guides.

An article entitled "ACR Appropriateness Criteria Headache" by Douglas and colleagues[48] in 2014 suggests that imaging may be "useful" for the following patients with headache: "…associated with trauma; new, worse, or abrupt onset; thunderclap; radiating to the neck; due to trigeminal autonomic cephalgia; persistent and positional; and temporal in older individuals." These investigators go on to also mention that "Pregnant patients, immunocompromised individuals, cancer patients, and patients with papilledema or systemic illnesses, including hypercoagulable disorders may benefit from imaging."[48]

Use of Guidelines

Young and colleagues[26] reported in 2018 that "An estimated 35% of patients were imaged against guidelines" in their study regarding outpatients with headache. An article published in 2015 by Rosenberg and colleagues[49] noted a decrease in imaging of patients with headache from 14.9% to 13.4% in their system, which was a statistically significant change; they attributed this change to Image Wisely. Thought-provokingly, Lester and Liu reminded us via an article in 2013 that "…value of negative imaging should not be underestimated in the cost-benefit analysis…"[1]

COMPUTED TOMOGRAPHY VERSUS MR IMAGING

When considering the choice of CT versus MR imaging, it is imperative to ensure that one can expect the clinical question to likely be answered with the chosen modality. If the clinical question cannot be expected to be answered sufficiently, it is characteristically the job of the Radiologist to suggest the more appropriate imaging examination, if one exists. To this end, excellent communication between referring providers and radiologists is essential to outstanding patient care. CT is typically more (geographically) available, faster, and cheaper. MR imaging typically provides more information. In the authors' experience, it is commonly said by nonradiologists that CT is superior to MR imaging at identification of intracranial hemorrhage; however, this has not been what they have found in their practice, at least anecdotally. That being said, time is usually of the essence when intracranial hemorrhage is suspected and in this setting CT is usually preferable.

For example, an MR imaging of the head with and without contrast material is a highly rated examination of choice (rating of 8 in ACR AC) in the setting of new-onset headache with focal neurologic deficit or papilledema.[2] On the other hand, a CT head with contrast has a lower rating of 5

but might be useful if MR imaging is not available or is contraindicated.[2]

Some investigators have communicated for a "two-tiered approach" to MR imaging including focused MR sequences as an approach to the cost-effective workup of patients with headache.[50]

An article by Douglas and colleagues[48] in 2014 about the ACR AC regarding headache notes that "Unlike most headaches, those associated with cough, exertion, or sexual activity usually required neuroimaging with MRI of the brain with and without contrast…"

A local approach to this is to promote CT if there is anything urgent, emergent, or acute about the clinical scenario and to promote MR imaging otherwise, if the patient may receive either examination. Advanced neuroimaging (eg, functional MR imaging or MR spectroscopy) is not usually helpful for the workup of headache in the setting of a normal conventional MR imaging. Anecdotally, the authors have also not found a benefit to use of 3 T MR imaging scanners over 1.5 T versions for the workup of uncomplicated headache. One way to optimize utilization of resources is to look for all of the already-made available diagnoses on the scans interpreted, especially noting those that may answer the clinical question, for example, imaging findings of an enlarged, partially empty sella and papilledema that may explain headache via idiopathic intracranial hypertension (Fig. 1). Overlooking diagnoses on neuroimaging of patients with headache that may explain the presentation but are not "acute intracranial pathology" is not a good use of resources. A few commonly (in our experience) overlooked diagnoses that may explain headache include intracranial increased or decreased pressure abnormalities, sinusitis, middle ear and/or mastoid air cell disease, and temporomandibular joint disease. Of note, contraindications, relative or absolute, may affect this decision-making process.

CONTRAST MATERIAL

The decision of whether or not to use contrast material for CT or MR imaging is another consideration when choosing the appropriate examination. For example, if a patient presents with a sudden onset of severe headache (eg, "worst headache of life"), a CT head without contrast is the preferred initial examination with an ACR AC rating of 9.[2] This step is usually crucial to search for subarachnoid hemorrhage, especially in the appropriate clinical setting. In contradistinction, CT scan of the head with contrast is given a rating of 3, ostensibly because the intravenous contrast could obscure subarachnoid hemorrhage.[2]

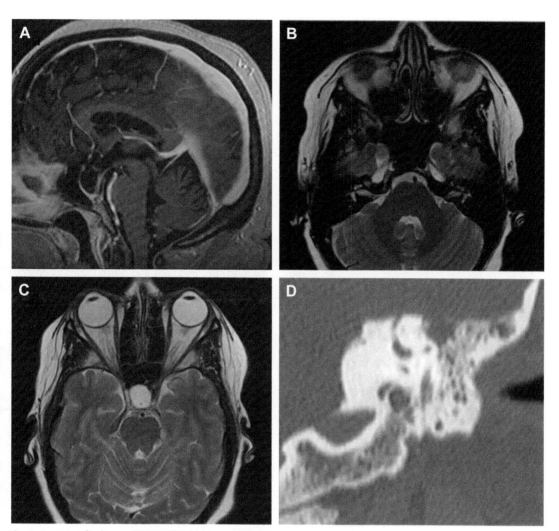

Fig. 1. Imaging findings of idiopathic intracranial hypertension. Sagittal T1-weighted postcontrast image (*A*) in a 26-year-old patient with headache due to idiopathic intracranial hypertension demonstrates an enlarged, partially empty sella. Axial T2 noncontrast images (*B*) in the same patient reveal enlargement of the Meckel cave bilaterally with a right-sided petrous apex meningocele and enlarged subarachnoid perioptic spaces bilaterally (*C*). Coronal bone-algorithm images of the left temporal bone (*D*) demonstrate thinning of the tegmen tympani with a small meningocele and dehiscence of the superior semicircular canal at the arcuate eminence.

A local approach to this is to promote noncontrast imaging in the absence of a clear indication for contrast material. Even when contrast material is indicated, the exclusion of noncontrast imaging is typically ill advised (please see the earlier discussion). One area in which contrast material administration is found to be particularly useful is with the identification of leptomeningeal processes on MR imaging, especially with postcontrast FLAIR images. Specialized contrast-enhanced examinations such as CT angiography (eg, to evaluate for aneurysm) and MR or CT venography (eg, to evaluate for venous sinus thrombosis) may be of clinical interest. In some instances, use of MR angiography (when used in patients with headache, presumably the primary concern is for aneurysm) may be preferable to contrast-enhanced MR imaging and/or CT with its ionizing radiation. As discussed earlier, contraindications, relative or absolute, may also affect this decision-making process.

SUMMARY

Headache is a common indication for neuroimaging. Attention to quality, safety, utilization, and appropriateness including attention to relevant socioeconomics should benefit these patients and the health care system. In addition to a plethora of scholarly articles, many guidelines serve as assets in the care of these patients. Consideration of imaging in patients presenting with headache is an important aspect of health care and familiarity with these concepts and resources should help.

ACKNOWLEDGMENTS

The authors would like to thank Dr Ryan Peterson for assistance with figure formatting.

REFERENCES

1. Lester MS, Liu BP. Imaging in the evaluation of headache. Med Clin North Am 2013;97(2):243–65.
2. Douglas AC, Wippold FJ 2nd, Broderick DF, et al. American College of radiology ACR appropriateness criteria: headache 2013. Available at: https://acsearch.acr.org/docs/69482/Narrative/. Accessed March 1, 2018.
3. Hainer BL, Matheson EM. Approach to acute headache in adults. Am Fam Physician 2013;87(10): 682–7.
4. WHO. Headache disorders 2016. Available at: http://www.who.int/en/news-room/fact-sheets/detail/headache-disorders. Accessed May 24, 2018.
5. Goldstein JN, Camargo CA Jr, Pelletier AJ, et al. Headache in United States emergency departments: demographics, work-up and frequency of pathological diagnoses. Cephalalgia 2006;26(6): 684–90.
6. Friedman BW, Serrano D, Reed M, et al. Use of the emergency department for severe headache. A population-based study. Headache 2009;49(1): 21–30.
7. Minen MT, Loder E, Friedman B. Factors associated with emergency department visits for migraine: an observational study. Headache 2014;54(10):1611–8.
8. Steiner TJ, Birbeck GL, Jensen R, et al. Lifting the burden: the first 7 years. J Headache Pain 2010; 11(6):451–5.
9. Steiner TJ, Birbeck GL, Jensen RH, et al. Headache disorders are third cause of disability worldwide. J Headache Pain 2015;16:58.
10. Global Burden of Disease Study Collaborators. Global, regional, and national incidence, prevalence, and years lived with disability for 301 acute and chronic diseases and injuries in 188 countries, 1990-2013: a systematic analysis for the Global Burden of Disease Study 2013. Lancet 2015; 386(9995):743–800.
11. Fitch K, Bernstein SJ, Aguilar MD, et al. The RAND/UCLA appropriateness method user's manual 2001. Available at: https://www.rand.org/pubs/monograph_reports/MR1269.html. Accessed July 04, 2018.
12. Hendee WR, Becker GJ, Borgstede JP, et al. Addressing overutilization in medical imaging. Radiology 2010;257(1):240–5.
13. Medicine Io. To err is human: building a safer health system. Washington (DC): The National Academies Press; 2000.
14. Strauss KJ, Kaste SC. The ALARA (as low as reasonably achievable) concept in pediatric interventional and fluoroscopic imaging: striving to keep radiation doses as low as possible during fluoroscopy of pediatric patients—a white paper executive summary. Radiology 2006;240(3):621–2.
15. Image gently. Available at: https://www.imagegently.org/. Accessed July 04, 2018.
16. Olesen J, Steiner T, Bousser MG, et al. Proposals for new standardized general diagnostic criteria for the secondary headaches. Cephalalgia 2009;29(12): 1331–6.
17. Clinch CR. Evaluation of acute headaches in adults. Am Fam Physician 2001;63(4):685–92.
18. Cady RK. Red flags and comfort signs for ominous secondary headaches. Otolaryngol Clin North Am 2014;47(2):289–99.
19. Ravishankar K. WHICH headache to investigate, WHEN, and HOW? Headache 2016;56(10):1685–97.
20. Grant R. Overview: brain tumour diagnosis and management/Royal College of Physicians guidelines. J Neurol Neurosurg Psychiatry 2004; 75(Suppl 2):ii18–23.
21. Porter KR, McCarthy BJ, Freels S, et al. Prevalence estimates for primary brain tumors in the United States by age, gender, behavior, and histology. Neuro Oncol 2010;12(6):520–7.
22. Rasmussen BK, Jensen R, Schroll M, et al. Epidemiology of headache in a general population–a prevalence study. J Clin Epidemiol 1991;44(11):1147–57.
23. Sobri M, Lamont AC, Alias NA, et al. Red flags in patients presenting with headache: clinical indications for neuroimaging. Br J Radiol 2003;76(908):532–5.
24. Dodick D. Diagnosing headache: clinical clues and clinical rules. Adv Stud Med 2003;3(2):87–92.
25. Nye BL, Ward TN. Clinic and emergency room evaluation and testing of headache. Headache 2015; 55(9):1301–8.
26. Young NP, Elrashidi MY, McKie PM, et al. Neuroimaging utilization and findings in headache outpatients: significance of red and yellow flags. Cephalalgia 2018;38(12):1841–8.
27. Foundation MR. Migraine facts 2018. Available at: http://migraineresearchfoundation.org/about-migraine/migraine-facts/. Accessed May 24, 2018.
28. Munakata J, Hazard E, Serrano D, et al. Economic burden of transformed migraine: results from the American Migraine Prevalence and Prevention (AMPP) Study. Headache 2009;49(4):498–508.
29. Stokes M, Becker WJ, Lipton RB, et al. Cost of health care among patients with chronic and episodic migraine in Canada and the USA: results from the International Burden of Migraine Study (IBMS). Headache 2011;51(7):1058–77.

30. Paul AB, Oklu R, Saini S, et al. How much is that head CT? Price transparency and variability in radiology. J Am Coll Radiol 2015;12(5):453–7.
31. Katz M. The cost-effective evaluation of uncomplicated headache. Med Clin North Am 2016;100(5):1009–17.
32. Vijayasarathi A, Hawkins CM, Hughes DR, et al. How Much do common imaging studies cost? a nationwide survey of radiology trainees. AJR Am J Roentgenol 2015;205(5):929–35.
33. Vijayasarathi A, Duszak R Jr, Gelbard RB, et al. Knowledge of the costs of diagnostic imaging: a survey of physician trainees at a Large Academic Medical Center. J Am Coll Radiol 2016;13(11):1304–10.
34. CAREOperative. Find your Fair price. Available at: https://www.healthcarebluebook.com/ui/consumerfront. Accessed May 24, 2018.
35. Larson EB, Omenn GS, Lewis H. Diagnostic evaluation of headache. Impact of computerized tomography and cost-effectiveness. JAMA 1980;243(4):359–62.
36. Mitchell CS, Osborn RE, Grosskreutz SR. Computed tomography in the headache patient: is routine evaluation really necessary? Headache 1993;33(2):82–6.
37. Akpek S, Arac M, Atilla S, et al. Cost-effectiveness of computed tomography in the evaluation of patients with headache. Headache 1995;35(4):228–30.
38. Holle D, Obermann M. The role of neuroimaging in the diagnosis of headache disorders. Ther Adv Neurol Disord 2013;6(6):369–74.
39. Evans RW. Diagnostic testing for the evaluation of headaches. Neurol Clin 1996;14(1):1–26.
40. Moeller JJ, Kurniawan J, Gubitz GJ, et al. Diagnostic accuracy of neurological problems in the emergency department. Can J Neurol Sci 2008;35(3):335–41.
41. Jordan YJ, Lightfoote JB, Jordan JE. Computed tomography imaging in the management of headache in the emergency department: cost efficacy and policy implications. J Natl Med Assoc 2009;101(4):331–5.
42. Silberstein SD. Practice parameter: evidence-based guidelines for migraine headache (an evidence-based review): report of the Quality Standards Subcommittee of the American Academy of Neurology. Neurology 2000;55(6):754–62.
43. Mitsikostas DD, Ashina M, Craven A, et al. European Headache Federation consensus on technical investigation for primary headache disorders. J Headache Pain 2015;17:5.
44. Kennis K, Kernick D, O'Flynn N. Diagnosis and management of headaches in young people and adults: NICE guideline. Br J Gen Pract 2013;63(613):443–5.
45. Morey SS. Headache Consortium releases guidelines for use of CT or MRI in migraine work-up. Am Fam Physician 2000;62(7):1699–701.
46. Sandrini G, Friberg L, Coppola G, et al. Neurophysiological tests and neuroimaging procedures in non-acute headache (2nd edition). Eur J Neurol 2011;18(3):373–81.
47. About the ACR appropriateness criteria. Available at: https://www.acr.org/Clinical-Resources/ACR-Appropriateness-Criteria/About-the-ACR-AC. Accessed July 05, 2018.
48. Douglas AC, Wippold FJ 2nd, Broderick DF, et al. ACR appropriateness criteria headache. J Am Coll Radiol 2014;11(7):657–67.
49. Rosenberg A, Agiro A, Gottlieb M, et al. Early trends among seven recommendations from the choosing wisely campaign. JAMA Intern Med 2015;175(12):1913–20.
50. Sharma A, Reis M, Parsons MS, et al. Two-tiered approach to MRI for headache: a cost-effective way to use an expensive technology. AJR Am J Roentgenol 2013;201(1):W75–80.

Intracranial Hypotension and Cerebrospinal Fluid Leak

Stephen M. Chan, MD[a], Yosef G. Chodakiewitz, MD[a],
Marcel M. Maya, MD[b], Wouter I. Schievink, MD[c],
Franklin G. Moser, MD, MMM[b],*

KEYWORDS

• CSF leak • Intracranial hypotension • Headache • Brain

KEY POINTS

• Intracranial hypotension can cause debilitating orthostatic pain and neurologic symptoms.
• Imaging findings can guide diagnosis with a high degree of confidence despite the varied clinical presentation.
• Treatment most often consists of targeted or nontargeted epidural injections, with surgical intervention reserved for patients with recurrent symptoms despite multiple targeted injections.

INTRODUCTION

Intracranial hypotension is an important cause of persistent headache that has gained increasing recognition over the past 20 years.[1–7] Patients typically present with orthostatic headache but can also experience a spectrum of neurologic symptoms ranging from nausea and blurry vision to dementia and coma.[8–10] Intracranial hypotension is typically caused by loss of cerebrospinal fluid (CSF) through a dural defect or CSF-venous fistula in the thoracic or lumbar spine, although the underlying pathophysiology remains incompletely understood.[11]

Recognition of intracranial hypotension has important implications for both patients and health care providers. The debilitating pain and neurologic symptoms associated with the condition can often be effectively treated by relatively noninvasive procedures. The biggest challenge is most often one of diagnosis, because of the wide range of possible symptoms with which these patients may present; however, imaging findings can guide the diagnosis with a high degree of confidence. Prompt recognition of intracranial hypotension can potentially help avoid a lengthy work-up or unnecessary invasive procedures.

Epidemiologic data are limited; however, incidence is estimated to be 5 per 100,000 based on a recent study of emergency room patients in an urban academic hospital.[12] Peak incidence occurs around 40 years of age, but it can affect patients of any age.[13] There is an increased prevalence in women, with a female/male ratio of 1.5:1. The major predisposing factor is a weakness in the dura, as seen in hereditary connective tissue disorders[14,15] (Fig. 1).

CLINICAL PRESENTATION

Typical presentation for intracranial hypotension is an orthostatic headache, worse in the upright

Disclosures: None.
[a] Cedars-Sinai Medical Center, 8700 Beverly Boulevard, Taper Building, Suite M335, Los Angeles, CA 90048, USA; [b] Cedars-Sinai Medical Center, 8700 Beverly Boulevard, South Tower, Suite 8517, Los Angeles, CA 90048, USA; [c] Cedars-Sinai Medical Center, Advanced Health Sciences Pavilion, Suite A6600, 127 South San Vicente Boulevard, Los Angeles, CA 90048, USA
* Corresponding author.
E-mail address: Franklin.moser@cshs.org

Neuroimag Clin N Am 29 (2019) 213–226
https://doi.org/10.1016/j.nic.2019.01.002

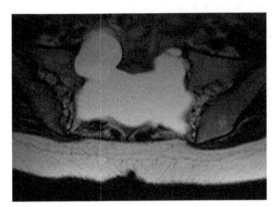

Fig. 1. Axial T2 magnetic resonance (MR) imaging of the lumbar spine showing dural ectasia in a patient with Marfan syndrome.

position. However, there is a wide-ranging time course of symptom onset, as it relates to the positional change. Symptom onset may occur within seconds of becoming upright, or not for hours; conversely, symptoms may improve within minutes of recumbency, or also not for hours.[1,2,6] The positional aspect of the headache itself can be variable and change with time, with some patients experiencing reversal of the normal orthostatic pattern. These variable characteristics have been attributed to physiologic compensation over time.[16] Additional associated symptoms have been reported and are summarized in Table 1.[9,10,16–22]

Intracranial hypotension from CSF leak can be spontaneous, iatrogenic, or traumatic. Spontaneous cases result from dural tears, meningeal diverticulum, or CSF-venous fistulas in the thoracic or lumbar spine.[5] Most so-called spontaneous cases have no clear precipitating event, but patients often recollect having had some otherwise trivial traumatic event before the initial onset of their symptoms, such as lifting small objects,

stretching, sports, roller coaster rides, and falls.[23] Iatrogenic CSF leaks can result from epidural injections, lumbar punctures, intrathecal catheters, or surgery.[21,24–26] Some CSF leaks have been attributed to obvious trauma, degenerative disc disease, or spinal osteophytes. Sometimes traumatic brachial plexus avulsions lead to intracranial hypotension.[27]

Dural weakness is the only known predisposing factor for intracranial hypotension and is primarily seen in hereditary disorders of connective tissue (HDCT). Studies have shown an increased incidence of intracranial hypotension, meningeal diverticula, and dural defects in patients with HDCT such as Marfans, Ehlers-Danlos, or adult polycystic kidney disease.[14,15] Other patients showing signs of underlying connective tissue disorders, such as history of lens dislocation, retinal detachment, or cardiac valve abnormalities, have also been reported to have higher incidence of intracranial hypotension.[28–31]

NORMAL ANATOMY, PHYSIOLOGY, AND IMAGING

CSF is contained within the cerebral ventricles, as well as within the cranial and spinal subarachnoid spaces. Normally, the mean total CSF volume is 150 mL, with 25 mL contained within the ventricles and the remaining 125 mL dispersed throughout the subarachnoid spaces. The traditional concept of CSF physiology is one of a secretion-circulation-absorption circuit, as follows.

Beginning in the cerebral ventricles, CSF gets predominantly secreted by the choroid plexuses into the ventricular spaces. CSF then flows in a rostrocaudal fashion through the ventricular system, and drains out into the subarachnoid spaces through foramina in the fourth ventricle; the medial foramen of Magendie facilitates fourth ventricular drainage into the cisterna magna,

Table 1 Symptoms of intracranial hypotension			
Generalized Symptoms	**Cranial Nerve Deficits**	**Spinal Manifestations**	**Severe Intracranial Manifestations**
Neck pain or stiffness	Blurry vision, visual field defects, diplopia	Back pain	Cognitive dysfunction
Nausea	Loss of balance	Radiculopathy	Dementia
Photophobia	Facial numbness or pain, facial weakness	Myelopathy	Parkinsonism
—	Phonophobia, muffled hearing, tinnitus	—	Ataxia
—	Dysgeusia	—	Stupor and coma

and the lateral foramina of Luschka enables drainage into the cerebellar-pontine angle cisterns. CSF then continues to flow in a multidirectional fashion through the cranial and spinal subarachnoid spaces to sites of absorption. Intracranially, subarachnoid CSF flows toward subarachnoid villi protruding in the dural venous sinuses, where CSF is absorbed into the blood; additional intracranial CSF absorption sites also include the olfactory mucosa and cranial nerve sheaths, which receive lymphatic drainage. Analogously, intraspinal subarachnoid CSF is partially absorbed at the spinal epidural plexus through spinal subarachnoid villi into the blood and is also partially absorbed by spinal nerve sheaths into the lymphatic system, whereas the remainder flows rostrally to participate in the intracranial subarachnoid absorption system just described.[32,33]

Historically, the essential function of CSF was proposed as a fluid cushion serving a hydromechanical protective role for the brain and spinal cord. Recent data from molecular biology support additional functional roles of CSF, showing that CSF plays essential roles in homeostasis of the molecular environment of the interstitial fluid of brain parenchyma and consequent regulation of neuronal functioning[32,33] (Table 2).

FINDINGS
Cranial Computed Tomography

Cranial computed tomography (CT) is often the first test obtained in an emergency setting for patients presenting with headache, neck pain, and nausea. Cranial CT is not particularly sensitive for intracranial hypotension but may show subdural fluid collections, downward displacement of the cerebellar tonsils, or effacement of the basal cisterns. Increased attenuation in the basal cisterns, sylvian fissures, and the tentorium are occasionally seen and can be mistaken for subarachnoid hemorrhage. Brain sagging and pachymeningeal enhancement on magnetic resonance (MR) imaging as well as lack of edema can be key in differentiating the two.[38]

Cranial Magnetic Resonance Imaging

Cranial MR is diagnostic of intracranial hypotension approximately 80% of the time. The main findings can be summarized with the mnemonic SEEPS:

1. Subdural fluid collections
2. Enhancement of the pachymeninges
3. Engorgement of venous structures
4. Pituitary hyperemia
5. Sagging of the brain

Table 2 Imaging protocols	
CT brain without contrast	• Most common first-line examination • Low sensitivity
MR imaging brain with contrast	• MR imaging obtained with intravenous gadolinium • Axial FLAIR, axial T2 turbo spin echo, axial susceptibility-weighted imaging, sagittal T2 spin echo, axial T1 MPR postcontrast • Shows findings of intracranial hypotension approximately 80% of the time[1]
CT myelogram	• Thin-cut CT of the spine with intrathecal iodinated contrast • Historical gold standard for detection and localization of spinal CSF leaks • Dynamic CT myelogram can be performed in various positions and with rapid repositioning to elucidate otherwise difficult-to-detect leaks
Spinal MR imaging	• Traditionally performed with intravenous gadolinium • Sagittal T1, sagittal T2, axial T2, and coronal T2 haste, with 3D and maximum intensity projection reconstructions • Heavily T2-weighted myelographic sequences have been shown to have similar sensitivity to CT myelogram in some studies[34] • Intrathecal gadolinium has been shown in some studies to increase sensitivity[35,36] • Intrathecal saline has also been shown to increase sensitivity[37]
Digital subtraction myelogram	• Digital subtraction fluoroscopy during intrathecal contrast injection • Often performed with anesthesia to remove respiratory motion artifact • Useful in localizing rapid leaks or CSF-venous fistulae not visualized on MR imaging or CT myelography[16]

Abbreviations: 3D. three-dimensional; FLAIR, fluid-attenuated inversion recovery; MPR, multiplanar reconstruction.

Subdural fluid collections are seen in approximately 36% of cases and most commonly consist of bilateral subdural hygromas at the frontal convexities.[2] Hematomas are also possible[39] (**Fig. 2**).

Enhancement of the pachymeninges is the most well-known and most common finding for intracranial hypotension, seen in up to 80% of patients.[40] Enhancement is most often diffuse involving the supratentorial and infratentorial meninges. A wavelike enhancement in the temporal pachymeninges has also been described[41] (**Fig. 3**).

Engorgement of the dural sinuses and cerebral veins is also a common but subtle finding. Despite its subtlety, 1 case series found it to have nearly 95% sensitivity and specificity.[42]

Pituitary hyperemia is a less common but more specific finding consisting of intense pituitary enhancement, sometimes mimicking an adenoma in appearance.[3]

Sagging of the brain is seen with effacement of perichiasmatic cisterns, bowing of the optic chiasm, flattening of the pituitary stalk and pons, effacement of the prepontine cisterns, and descent of the cerebellar tonsils. Although the presence of subdural collections and descent of the cerebellar tonsils may suggest cerebellar herniation secondary to mass effect from the subdural collections, in intracranial hypotension the degree of cerebellar downward displacement is generally out of proportion to the mass effect caused by these collections; the subdural

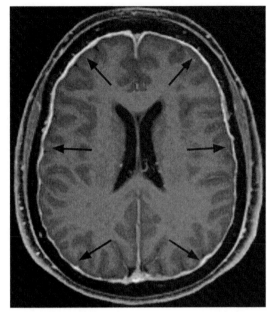

Fig. 3. T1 postcontrast cranial MR imaging showing pachymeningeal thickening and enhancement (*arrows*) in a patient with intracranial hypotension.

collections are caused by the downward descent and negative pressure, rather than vice versa. If a misinterpretation leads to an overzealous interventional drainage of the subdural collections, this could exacerbate the problem in intracranial hypotension[43] (**Fig. 4**).

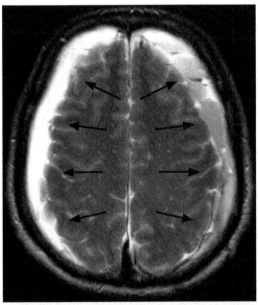

Fig. 2. Axial T2 cranial MR imaging showing bilateral extradural fluid collections (*arrows*) in a patient with intracranial hypotension.

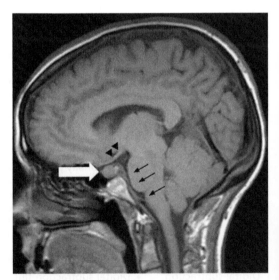

Fig. 4. Sagittal T1 cranial MR imaging showing sagging of the midbrain with pituitary engorgement (*white arrow*), bowing of the optic chiasm (*arrowheads*), and effacement of the pons (*black arrows*) in a patient with intracranial hypotension.

In a recent unpublished series, edema of the corticospinal tracts in the midbrain was described as a novel finding. In this series, 55% of patients with intracranial hypotension had associated MR signal changes in the midbrain corticospinal tracts consistent with edema, compared with no such changes seen in a control group of patients with nonorthostatic headache.[43] Among the patients with intracranial hypotension, the presence of edema was correlated with diminished mamillo-pontine distance, potentially reflecting degree of midbrain distortion and possibly portending worse outcomes. Causes of the edema have been speculated to be possibly secondary to long-standing compression, or possibly secondary to injury of axons within the midbrain caused by stretching along their axes[43] (Fig. 5).

Sometimes seen in intracranial hypotension is superficial siderosis, a condition in which hemosiderin is deposited on the pial surface of the brain and/or spinal cord, typically as a result of chronic bleeding in the subarachnoid space. Superficial siderosis is best detected on gradient-recalled echo or susceptibility-weighted MR imaging. The superficial siderosis seen in intracranial hypotension is speculated as secondary to recurrent bleeding from superior cerebellar bridging veins that are stretched because of brain sagging or intraspinal hemorrhage from friable vessels. The typical scenario in which superficial siderosis is seen in intracranial hypotension is that of a patient who has symptoms of intracranial hypotension that remain untreated and is then eventually found to have superficial siderosis and a typically ventral spinal CSF leak on MR imaging years later[43] (Fig. 6).

Computed Tomography Myelogram

CT myelogram has long been considered the gold standard for identifying and localizing CSF leaks.[16,44] The most common finding is an extradural fluid collection. In some cases, contrast extravasation at the site of the leak can be directly visualized. Adjusting CT timing based on leak speed, with brisk leaks receiving prompt imaging and slow leaks delayed imaging, can increase leak detection and localization.[6] Dynamic CT myelogram can also be performed, with intrathecal contrast injection during CT imaging. Such techniques can be performed with rapid patient repositioning between scans to elucidate small ventral leaks or those associated with nerve root sleeves.[44] It should be noted that a posterior spinal fluid collection at C1 to C2 is a known false-localizing sign seen in up 10% of patients.[45]

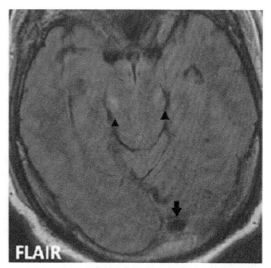

FLAIR

Fig. 5. Axial fluid-attenuated inversion recovery (FLAIR) cranial MR imaging showing corticospinal tract edema (*arrowheads*) and dural sinus engorgement (*arrow*) in a patient with intracranial hypotension.

Spinal Magnetic Resonance Imaging

Traditional spinal MR imaging can show meningeal enhancement, meningeal diverticula, extradural fluid collections, and dilated venous structures. MR imaging myelogram performed using heavily T2-weighted myelographic sequences or intrathecal gadolinium can localize leaks with similar sensitivity to CT myelography.[34,46] Intrathecal saline infusion has also been shown to improve sensitivity of leak detection by artificially increasing intrathecal pressure[35-37] (Fig. 7).

DIGITAL SUBTRACTION MYELOGRAM

Digital subtraction myelography (DSM) offers increased sensitivity for CSF leak detection. DSM is performed while the patient is under general endotracheal anesthesia with deep paralysis, because the technique involves controlled suspended respiration for maximal detail and temporal resolution. The patient is typically positioned prone in a biplane angiography suite with tilt-table capability. After a fluoroscopically guided lumbar puncture is performed and opening pressure obtained, the patient is repositioned based on the area of interest. In addition, contrast is manually injected (at a rate of approximately 1 mL/s) while also suspending the patient's respiration for 40 to 60 seconds; biplane subtraction images are simultaneously acquired at a rate of 2 to 3 frames/s.

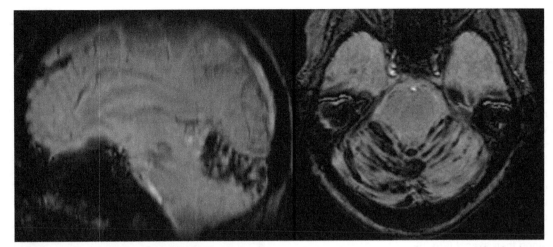

Fig. 6. Sagittal (*left*) and axial (*right*) susceptibility-weighted cranial MR imaging showing superficial siderosis affecting the cerebellum in a patient with intracranial hypotension.

In approximately half of cases, traditional CT myelography fails to localize the site of CSF leak. A direct fistulous connection between CSF and paraspinal veins has recently been recognized as a cause of CT myelogram–occult CSF leak in a subgroup of such cases.[47] A novel subtle imaging finding was recently described, known as the hyperdense paraspinal vein sign, which may assist in CSF-venous fistula identification, and consequently the site of CSF leak, in this subgroup of cases secondary to CSF-venous fistula. Giving rise to the name of this finding, a recent series described identification, on post-myelographic CT, of a hyperattenuated paraspinal vein in close proximity to the site of a CSF fistula that was ultimately identified at surgery. The hyperdense paraspinal vein sign presumably represents rapid passage of myelographic contrast into the venous system through the fistula. The correlate of this finding on digital subtraction myelogram is an opacified paraspinal vein, which is often more readily identified on digital subtraction myelogram. Recognition of this subtle finding may help localize the leak site in

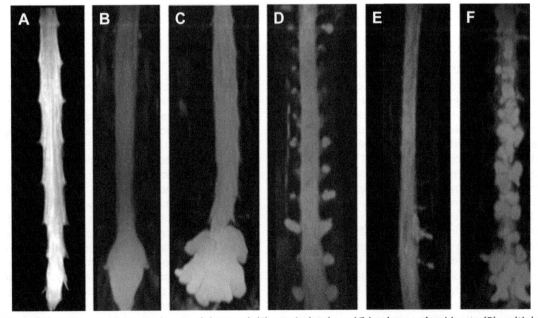

Fig. 7. MR imaging myelograms showing (*A*) normal, (*B*) ectatic dural sac, (*C*) lumbar arachnoid cysts, (*D*) multiple spinal arachnoid cysts, (*E*) small lumbar arachnoid cysts, (*F*) multiple focal dural ectasia with formation of saccules.

this subgroup of otherwise myelogram-occult CSF leak.[48,49]

DSM was formerly reserved for use in high-volume CSF leaks, which benefit from the real-time imaging capability of DSM, compared with the inherent time delay involved in postmyelogram CT. In these rapid leaks, by the time CT is performed, the contrast often has already spread over many levels and the exact site of the dural tear remains unknown. At our institution, we have expanded use of DSM to detect and localize CSF leak beyond just those with high-volume leaks. We now perform DSM in nearly all patients requiring leak detection and localization for targeted treatment, because in our experience it offers increased sensitivity for ventral leaks CSF venous fistulas and offers superior localization capabilities in detecting the site of dural defect[34,50,51] (Figs. 8–11).

DIAGNOSTIC CRITERIA

Diagnostic criteria for intracranial hypotension provided in the International Classification of Headache Disorders, Third Edition (ICHD-3), are listed later. Current criteria require low CSF pressure, imaged CSF leak, or typical brain MR imaging findings for diagnosis.

International Classification of Headache Disorders, Third Edition

A. Headache fulfilling criteria for 7.2 headache attributed to low CSF pressure, and criterion C below
B. Absence of a procedure or trauma known to be able to cause CSF leakage
C. Headache has developed in temporal relation to occurrence of low CSF pressure or CSF leakage, or has led to its discovery
D. Not better accounted for by another ICHD-3 diagnosis

Criteria 7.2

A. Any headache fulfilling criterion C
B. Either or both of the following:

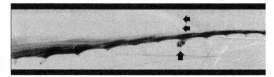

Fig. 8. Right lateral decubitus digital subtraction myelogram showing an opacified tangle of vessels and paraspinal vein (*arrows*), showing a CSF-venous fistula.

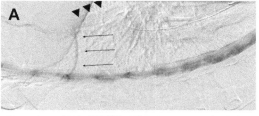

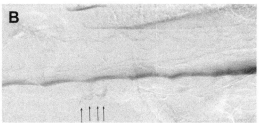

Fig. 9. Left lateral decubitus digital subtraction myelogram from the same patient. (*A*) Lateral series showing an opacified paraspinal vein (*arrows*) draining into the inferior vena cava (*arrowheads*); (*B*) frontal series showing opacification of a left paraspinal vein (*arrows*).

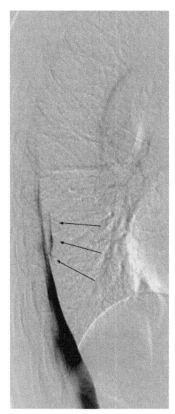

Fig. 10. Digital subtraction myelogram in the prone position showing a ventral CSF leak (*arrows*).

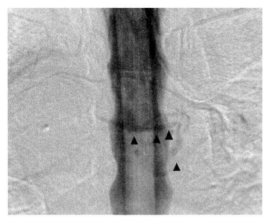

Fig. 11. Digital subtraction myelogram showing an opacified paraspinal vein (*arrowheads*) in a patient with a CSF-venous fistula.

    a. Low CSF pressure (<60 mm H_2O)
    b. Evidence of CSF leakage on imaging[a]
C. Headache has developed in temporal relation to the low CSF pressure or CSF leakage, or led to its discovery
D. Not better accounted for by another ICHD-3 diagnosis

However, the manifestations of intracranial hypotension are highly variable and many patients fail to satisfy the ICHD-3 criteria. A separate set of criteria has also been proposed, which also includes criteria for cranial MR imaging findings.[52] These criteria provide diagnosis for patients with normal CSF pressure (up to 60%[53]) or absent CSF leak on spinal imaging (up to 17%[2]).

1. Orthostatic headache
2. The presence of at least 1 of the following:
    a. Low opening pressure (60 mm H_2O)
    b. Sustained improvement of symptoms after epidural blood patching
    c. Demonstration of an active spinal CSF leak
    d. Cranial MR imaging changes of intracranial hypotension (eg, brain sagging or pachymeningeal enhancement)
3. No recent history of dural puncture
4. Not attributable to another disorder

CURRENT CLINICAL MANAGEMENT

The CSF leak/intracranial hypotension syndrome has historically been misdiagnosed and is a potentially complex clinical problem to effi-ciently approach, both diagnostically and therapeutically. The following approach may serve as a guideline for approaching the management of patients whose clinical presentation raises the clinical suspicion for intracranial hypotension and CSF leak.

Starting with the patient's initial presentation, suspicion of CSF leak is raised by the presence of a characteristic constellation of history, symptoms, and signs (eg, most commonly chronic orthostatic headache, possibly with other associated symptoms and perhaps in the setting of trivial trauma). MR imaging brain with and without contrast can subsequently be conducted to confirm the clinical suspicion, which has been shown to provide the diagnosis in 80% of cases.[16] If the MR imaging shows findings consistent with intracranial hypotension, the diagnosis can be considered confirmed and first-line treatment options may be offered; initial treatment options include either (1) an epidural blood patch procedure, or (2) conservative measures such as bed rest, oral/intravenous hydration, use of an abdominal binder, and generous caffeine intake. Because it is suspected that some unknown percentage of spontaneous CSF leaks resolve spontaneously without intervention, the conservative option is reasonable, particularly for uncomplicated presentations; however, in cases involving more complicated presentations (eg, chronic duration of symptoms, severe headache or disabling symptoms, aggressive precipitating injury, associated connective tissue disease, or hypermobility), it is our experience that purely conservative measures should not be expected to offer substantial or durable benefit.[16]

Epidural blood patching (EBP) is performed by injecting the patient's own blood through an epidural needle into the epidural space; it is not necessary to locally target the injection to the specific CSF leak site, and the injection is therefore typically administered simply in the lumbar region regardless of leak site in a nontargeted fashion with the patient in the Trendelenburg position. The therapeutic mechanism of action for EBP is incompletely understood but is likely multifactorial: (1) initially the injection of the fluid volume epidurally likely compresses the thecal sac to immediately increase lumbar and intracranial CSF pressure, and (2) the injected blood can clot over the CSF leak site and initiate an inflammatory

---

[a]Brain imaging showing brain sagging or pachymeningeal enhancement, or spine imaging (spine MR imaging, or MR imaging, CT, or DSM) showing extradural CSF.

reaction that facilitates healing at the puncture or leak site.

A substantial percentage of patients with CSF leak respond to epidural blood patch treatments; therefore, the option can be offered to patients once the diagnosis of intracranial hypotension has been confirmed by brain MR imaging, even if dedicated spinal imaging has been deferred or no specific CSF leak site has yet been identified.[16] In addition, EBP may be offered in cases with negative brain MR imaging when clinical suspicion for a CSF leak syndrome remains high, because 20% of intracranial hypotension cases may still go undetected after the initial brain MR imaging.[1] In those MR imaging–occult cases, the patient response after EBP may itself offer diagnostic information, with the diagnosis being supported if the patient obtains symptomatic relief.

EBP injection volumes range from small (10 mL) to large (100 mL), although the initial EBP trial is typically limited to small volumes of 10 to 20 mL of autologous blood injected. In patients that do not respond initially, or for those who responded but experience relapsing symptoms, the larger-volume EBP is recommended.[16] The authors usually perform larger-volume EBP via injections at 2 levels, one at the thoracolumbar junction and a second at a lower lumbar level, with the maximum volume of injected blood varying according to the limit from resulting local or radicular pain in the patient. When several EBPs are required, repeat procedures are spaced out by a minimum of 5 days in between.[16]

When even repeat EBP fails to provide adequate relief symptomatic relief, the next line of treatments involves targeted interventions, requiring specific characterization and anatomic localization of the CSF leak site from the spine. The various dedicated spine imaging modalities described earlier can be of value, each offering varying strengths and shortcomings. Once the CSF leak site can be precisely identified, an appropriate targeted intervention can be offered. Historically, when nontargeted EBP failed to offer relief to patients, the next alternative was invasive surgery to directly repair the dural defect in the operating room. However, some leak sites may be amenable to a percutaneous approach via fluoroscopic or CT-guided epidural patching with injection of fibrin sealant directly to the confirmed leak site, and ought to be considered and potentially offered to patients as a less invasive therapeutic option that can be achieved in the outpatient setting and potentially obviate open surgery[54] (Fig. 12).

However, when the location or type of CSF leak is not amenable to a targeted percutaneous approach, or when a targeted fibrin sealant injection also fails, a surgical option must be considered. The specific procedure is tailored to the individual, depending on the specific anatomy, location of the spinal CSF leak, and CSF leak type. Posterior CSF leaks and leaks along nerve roots are often, although not always, easier to access surgically from a posterior approach; the approach for ventral leaks is evolving. At present, the authors approach ventral leaks at the cervical level with corpectomy and discectomy, ventral thoracic leaks with a transdural and transpedicular approach, and ventral lumbar leaks with a direct approach between the nerve roots.[16] In addition, a recently described classification system, for cases of spontaneous intracranial hypotension, to differentiate CSF leaks into 4 separate types may help guide the most appropriate surgical planning[5] (Fig. 13).

Type 1 leaks consist of a dural tear and are almost always associated with an extradural CSF collection. Type 1 leaks can be further subdivided into type 1a leaks, representing ventral CSF leaks; and type 1b leaks, representing posterolateral CSF leaks. At surgery, type 1 leaks have been described as invariably vertically oriented along the fibers of the dura.[5] The dural tears in type 1 leaks are usually related to an injury to the dura

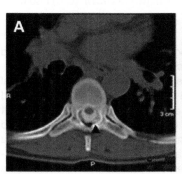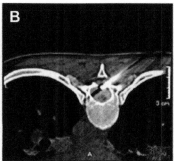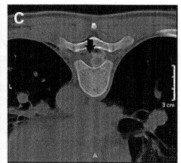

Fig. 12. (A) Preprocedural CT myelogram of a thoracic CSF leak (*arrowhead*), (B) CT-guided fibrin glue injection, (C) postprocedural CT showing fibrin glue filling defect at the site of the leak (*arrow*).

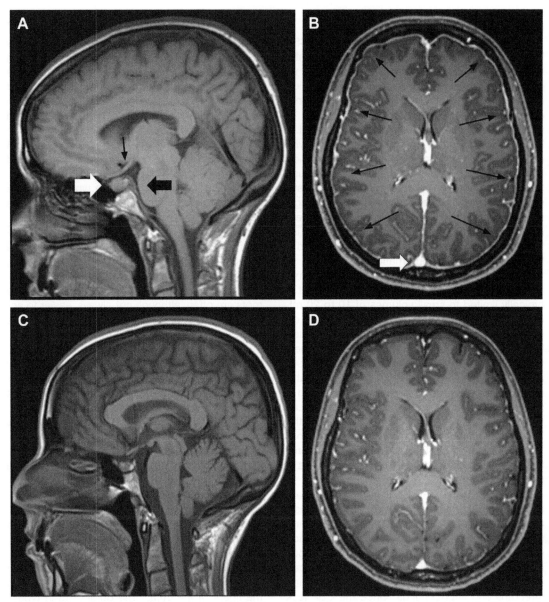

Fig. 13. Pretreatment and posttreatment cranial MR images showing (*A*) pituitary engorgement (*white arrow*), bowing of the optic chiasm (*small black arrow*), and effacement of the pons (*large black arrow*); (*B*) pachymeningeal thickening and enhancement (*black arrows*) and venous sinus engorgement (*white arrow*); (*C, D*) resolution of intracranial hypotension–related findings.

from an adjacent bony abnormality or some calcification at the level of the disc space.

Our surgical approach to type 1 involves identifying the dural tear under microscopic epidural inspection around the spinal cord. Once identified, the tear can be directly repaired with sutures. However, if the dura is too weak or friable to be adequately sutured or if the tear is too medial to be safely directly sutured from a posterior approach, we have placed a small muscle graft around the tear to achieve the closure. We have had equivalent

success with both the direct suture technique and muscle graft technique in these cases.

Type 2 leaks consist of significant meningeal diverticula (>8 mm), and are also subdivided into types 2a and 2b. Type 2a leaks represent simple single or multiple diverticula. Type 2b leaks represent complex meningeal diverticula or dural ectasia.[5] Dedicated spinal imaging confirms the diverticula to be the demonstrable leak source of an extradural CSF collection in only about 20% of cases; however, in some of

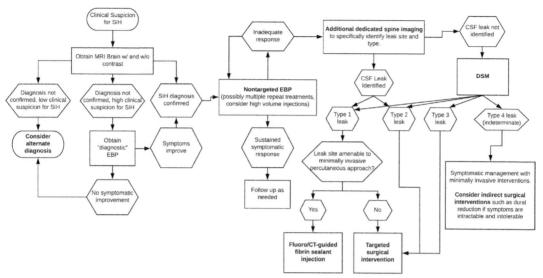

Fig. 14. Clinical management algorithm. SIH, spontaneous intracranial hypotension.

those patients with imaging-occult leaks who nevertheless go on to surgery, it has been reported that, at surgery, CSF is nevertheless sometimes still seen seeping through the thin lining of those diverticula.[5] In some type 2 cases, the meningeal diverticula may be responsible for spontaneous intracranial hypotension through the process of CSF pooling within the dilated dural sacs rather than CSF leakage.[5] The surgical treatment of these spinal meningeal diverticula directed at the largest, most irregular cysts is often successful in the treatment of spontaneous intracranial hypotension. The authors have found the use of small titanium aneurysm clips to be effective in sealing off the targeted diverticula. Sometimes, in cases in which a specific diverticular leak site or hole can be identified, and the dura is of a good quality, we have also used direct suturing or small muscle grafts to directly repair the leak in these cases. Other times, particularly in cases of dural ectasia, we have had success coating the dura with artificial dura graft that seals to the patient's own dura over a period of a month.

Type 3 CSF leaks consist of the direct CSF-venous fistulas. These patients never show an associated extradural CSF collection on dedicated spinal imaging. At surgery, these fistulas can consist of a single draining venous channel or of a network of dilated veins surrounding the spinal nerve root sleeve.[5] The authors have had promising results treating these types of leak by using small titanium clips to interrupt the fistula or by using small electrocautery to obliterate the venous channel.

Type 4 CSF leaks describe the remainder of leak types without a confirmed source on any dedicated spinal imaging modality and that remain otherwise indeterminate as to type. Among type 4 leaks, there is an extradural CSF collection in approximately 50% of cases, whereas in the remaining half there is no demonstrable evidence of extradural CSF. The authors have rarely performed surgery in these types of patients without a specifically identifiable surgical target. However, in a small cohort of type-4 patients with intolerable symptoms of intracranial hypotension that remain intractable to less invasive interventions, we have attempted some novel surgical interventions for indirect treatments that have provided some benefit. These indirect surgical interventions have included lumbar dural reduction surgery, in which a lumbar laminectomy is performed, a strip of dura is resected, and the dural defect is closed; the resulting decrease in lumbar CSF volume is thought to increase intracranial CSF volume and pressure.[55] It has also been shown that infusion of saline into the epidural space may offer symptomatic benefit, and we have a small cohort of patients who have achieved some symptomatic benefit from implantation of an epidural catheter with subcutaneous port for regular infusions of saline[16] (**Fig. 14**).

DIFFERENTIAL DIAGNOSIS

- Meningitis
- Pituitary adenoma
- Meningeal metastases
- Postsurgical dural thickening

- Chronic subdural hematoma
- Dural sinus thrombosis
- Postural orthostatic tachycardia syndrome

PEARLS, PITFALLS, VARIANTS

- Although cranial CSF leaks cause a loss of CSF, they do not cause intracranial hypotension. Symptomatic patients should be evaluated for spinal CSF leaks.[45]
- False localizing sign of C1-2: retrospinal fluid collection at C1-2, seen in approximately 10% of patients.[45]
- Pseudosubarachnoid hemorrhage: consider intracranial hypotension with increased attenuation in the basal cisterns, sylvian fissure, and at the tentorium.[56]
- Meningeal diverticula or dilated nerve root sleeve are frequent sites of spontaneous CSF leaks.[57]

WHAT TREATING PHYSICIANS NEED TO KNOW

- Localization
- Leak classification
- Nearby spinal degenerative changes

SUMMARY

Prompt recognition and diagnosis of intracranial hypotension is important. Variable symptoms require an appropriately heightened index of clinical suspicion to initiate the appropriate imaging studies to make a timely diagnosis and subsequently provide treatment. Cranial MR imaging can provide diagnosis in 80% of cases but is normal in 20% of cases. The telltale constellation of signs on brain MR imaging of intracranial hypotension can by summarized using the mnemonic SEEPS (subdural fluid collections, enhancement of the pachymeninges, engorgement of venous structures, pituitary hyperemia, and sagging of the brain). Treatment is often an epidural blood patch intervention. When blood patches and conservative measures fail, careful localization of the CSF leak site is paramount to enable targeted intervention, via targeted blood or glue injection, or surgically to repair the dural defect.

REFERENCES

1. Schievink WI. Spontaneous spinal cerebrospinal fluid leaks and intracranial hypotension. JAMA 2006;295(19):2286–96.
2. Schievink WI. Spontaneous spinal cerebrospinal fluid leaks. Cephalalgia 2008;28(12):1345–56.
3. Mokri B. Spontaneous low pressure, low CSF volume headaches: spontaneous CSF leaks. Headache 2013;53(7):1034–53.
4. Mokri B. Spontaneous CSF leaks: low CSF volume syndromes. Neurol Clin 2014;32(2):397–422.
5. Schievink WI, Maya MM, Jean-Pierre S, et al. A classification system of spontaneous spinal CSF leaks. Neurology 2016;87(7):673–9.
6. Graff-Radford SB, Schievink WI. High-pressure headaches, low-pressure syndromes, and CSF leaks: diagnosis and management. Headache 2014;54(2):394–401.
7. Gordon RE, Moser FG, Pressman BD, et al. Resolution of pachymeningeal enhancement following dural puncture and blood patch. Neuroradiology 1995;37(7):557–8.
8. Kashmere JL, Jacka MJ, Emery D, et al. Reversible coma: a rare presentation of spontaneous intracranial hypotension. Can J Neurol Sci 2004;31(4):565–8.
9. Schievink WI, Moser FG, Pikul BK. Reversal of coma with an injection of glue. Lancet 2007;369(9570):1402.
10. Schievink WI, Maya MM, Barnard ZR, et al. Behavioral variant frontotemporal dementia as a serious complication of spontaneous intracranial hypotension. Oper Neurosurg (Hagerstown) 2018;15(5):505–15.
11. Schievink WI, Schwartz MS, Maya MM, et al. Lack of causal association between spontaneous intracranial hypotension and cranial cerebrospinal fluid leaks. J Neurosurg 2012;116(4):749–54.
12. Schievink WI, Maya MM, Moser F, et al. Frequency of spontaneous intracranial hypotension in the emergency department. J Headache Pain 2007;8(6):325–8.
13. Schievink WI, Maya MM, Louy C, et al. Spontaneous intracranial hypotension in childhood and adolescence. J Pediatr 2013;163(2):504–10.
14. Schievink WI, Gordon OK, Tourje J. Connective tissue disorders with spontaneous spinal cerebrospinal fluid leaks and intracranial hypotension: a prospective study. Neurosurgery 2004;54(1):65–70 [discussion: 70–1].
15. Reinstein E, Pariani M, Bannykh S, et al. Connective tissue spectrum abnormalities associated with spontaneous cerebrospinal fluid leaks: a prospective study. Eur J Hum Genet 2013;21(4):386–90.
16. Schievink WI, Deline CR. Headache secondary to intracranial hypotension. Curr Pain Headache Rep 2014;18(11):457.
17. Mokri B. Movement disorders associated with spontaneous CSF leaks: a case series. Cephalalgia 2014;34(14):1134–41.
18. Schievink WI, Maya MM. Quadriplegia and cerebellar hemorrhage in spontaneous intracranial hypotension. Neurology 2006;66(11):1777–8.

19. Tsai PH, Wang SJ, Lirng JF, et al. Spontaneous intra-cranial hypotension presenting as mental deterioration. Headache 2005;45(1):76–80.

20. Wicklund MR, Mokri B, Drubach DA, et al. Fronto-temporal brain sagging syndrome: an SIH-like presentation mimicking FTD. Neurology 2011;76(16): 1377–82.

21. Schievink WI, Palestrant D, Maya MM, et al. Spontaneous spinal cerebrospinal fluid leak as a cause of coma after craniotomy for clipping of an unruptured intracranial aneurysm. J Neurosurg 2009;110(3): 521–4.

22. Schievink WI, Maya MM, Moser FG, et al. Coma: a serious complication of spontaneous intracranial hypotension. Neurology 2018;90(19):e1638–45.

23. Schievink WI, Ebersold MJ, Atkinson JL. Roller-coaster headache due to spinal cerebrospinal fluid leak. Lancet 1996;347:1409.

24. Tu A, Creedon K, Sahjpaul R. Iatrogenic cerebrospinal fluid leak and intracranial hypotension after gynecological surgery. J Neurosurg Spine 2014; 21(3):450–3.

25. Lee CJ, Shim SM, Cho SH, et al. Iatrogenic development of cerebrospinal fluid leakage in diagnosing spontaneous intracranial hypotension. Korean J Fam Med 2018;39(2):122–5.

26. Schievink WI, Louy C. Precipitating factors of spontaneous spinal CSF leaks and intracranial hypotension. Neurology 2007;69(7):700–2.

27. Hebert-Blouin MN, Mokri B, Shin AY, et al. Cerebrospinal fluid volume-depletion headaches in patients with traumatic brachial plexus injury. J Neurosurg 2013;118(1):149–54.

28. Schievink WI, Maya MM. Frequency of intracranial aneurysms in patients with spontaneous intracranial hypotension. J Neurosurg 2011;115(1):113–5.

29. Schievink WI, Raissi SS. Spontaneous intracranial hypotension in patients with bicuspid aortic valve. J Heart Valve Dis 2012;21(6):714–7.

30. Pimienta AL, Rimoin DL, Pariani M, et al. Echocardiographic findings in patients with spontaneous CSF leak. J Neurol 2014;261(10):1957–60.

31. Schrijver I, Schievink WI, Godfrey M, et al. Spontaneous spinal cerebrospinal fluid leaks and minor skeletal features of Marfan syndrome: a microfibrill-opathy. J Neurosurg 2002;96(3):483–9.

32. Sakka L, Coll G, Chazal J. Anatomy and physiology of cerebrospinal fluid. Eur Ann Otorhinolaryngol Head Neck Dis 2011;128(6):309–16.

33. Brinker T, Stopa E, Morrison J, et al. A new look at cerebrospinal fluid circulation. Fluids Barriers CNS 2014;11:10.

34. Schievink WI. Novel neuroimaging modalities in the evaluation of spontaneous cerebrospinal fluid leaks. Curr Neurol Neurosci Rep 2013;13(7):358.

35. Chazen JL, Talbott JF, Lantos JE, et al. MR myelography for identification of spinal CSF leak in spontaneous intracranial hypotension. AJNR Am J Neuroradiol 2014;35(10):2007–12.

36. Akbar JJ, Luetmer PH, Schwartz KM, et al. The role of MR myelography with intrathecal gadolinium in localization of spinal CSF leaks in patients with spontaneous intracranial hypotension. AJNR Am J Neuroradiol 2012;33(3):535–40.

37. Griauzde J, Gemmete JJ, Pandey AS, et al. Intrathecal preservative-free normal saline challenge magnetic resonance myelography for the identification of cerebrospinal fluid leaks in spontaneous intracranial hypotension. J Neurosurg 2015;123(3):732–6.

38. Ferrante E, Regna-Gladin C, Arpino I, et al. Pseudo-subarachnoid hemorrhage: a potential imaging pitfall associated with spontaneous intracranial hypotension. Clin Neurol Neurosurg 2013;115(11): 2324–8.

39. Ferrante E, Rubino F, Beretta F, et al. Treatment and outcome of subdural hematoma in patients with spontaneous intracranial hypotension: a report of 35 cases. Acta Neurol Belg 2017; 118(1):61–70.

40. Schoffer KL, Benstead TJ, Grant I. Spontaneous intracranial hypotension in the absence of magnetic resonance imaging abnormalities. Can J Neurol Sci 2002;29(3):253–7.

41. Antony J, Hacking C, Jeffree RL. Pachymeningeal enhancement—a comprehensive review of literature. Neurosurg Rev 2015;38(4):649–59.

42. Farb RI, Forghani R, Lee SK, et al. The venous distension sign: a diagnostic sign of intracranial hypotension at MR imaging of the brain. AJNR Am J Neuroradiol 2007;28(8):1489–93.

43. Azizyan A, Smorodinsky E, Schievink W, et al. Corticospinal tract edema in the midbrain: a novel MR finding in patients with intracranial hypotension. Paper presented at: American Society of Neuroradiology 2015; Chicago, Illinois.

44. Kranz PG, Luetmer PH, Diehn FE, et al. Myelographic techniques for the detection of spinal CSF leaks in spontaneous intracranial hypotension. AJR Am J Roentgenol 2016;206(1):8–19.

45. Schievink WI, Maya MM, Chu RM, et al. False localizing sign of cervico-thoracic CSF leak in spontaneous intracranial hypotension. Neurology 2015; 84(24):2445–8.

46. Wang YF, Lirng JF, Fuh JL, et al. Heavily T2-weighted MR myelography vs CT myelography in spontaneous intracranial hypotension. Neurology 2009; 73(22):1892–8.

47. Schievink WI, Moser FG, Maya MM. CSF-venous fistula in spontaneous intracranial hypotension. Neurology 2014;83(5):472–3.

48. Kranz PG, Amrhein TJ, Schievink WI, et al. The "hyperdense paraspinal vein" sign: a marker of CSF-venous fistula. AJNR Am J Neuroradiol 2016;37(7): 1379–81.

49. Clark MS, Diehn FE, Verdoorn JT, et al. Prevalence of hyperdense paraspinal vein sign in patients with spontaneous intracranial hypotension without dural CSF leak on standard CT myelography. Diagn Interv Radiol 2018;24(1):54–9.

50. Schievink WI, Moser FG, Maya MM, et al. Digital subtraction myelography for the identification of spontaneous spinal CSF-venous fistulas. J Neurosurg Spine 2016;24(6):960–4.

51. Schievink WI, Maya MM, Moser FG. Digital subtraction myelography in the investigation of post-dural puncture headache in 27 patients: technical note. J Neurosurg Spine 2017;26(6):760–4.

52. Schievink WI, Dodick DW, Mokri B, et al. Diagnostic criteria for headache due to spontaneous intracranial hypotension: a perspective. Headache 2011; 51(9):1442–4.

53. Kranz PG, Tanpitukpongse TP, Choudhury KR, et al. How common is normal cerebrospinal fluid pressure in spontaneous intracranial hypotension? Cephalalgia 2016;36(13):1209–17.

54. Schievink WI, Maya MM, Moser FM. Treatment of spontaneous intracranial hypotension with percutaneous placement of a fibrin sealant: report of four cases. J Neurosurg 2004;100(6): 1098–100.

55. Schievink WI. A novel technique for treatment of intractable spontaneous intracranial hypotension: lumbar dural reduction surgery. Headache 2009; 49(7):1047–51.

56. Schievink WI, Maya MM, Tourje J, et al. Pseudo-subarachnoid hemorrhage: a CT-finding in spontaneous intracranial hypotension. Neurology 2005;65(1): 135–7.

57. Schievink WI, Maya MM. Spinal meningeal diverticula, spontaneous intracranial hypotension, and superficial siderosis. Neurology 2017;88(9): 916–7.

Headache Caused by Sinus Disease

Claudia F.E. Kirsch, MD*

KEYWORDS

- Migraine • Sinusitis • Autonomic dysfunction • Trigeminovascular pathway
- Low-dose computed axial tomography • Magnetic resonance imaging

KEY POINTS

- Headaches and sinus disease are common reasons to seek medical care; symptoms are similar and may relate to autonomic dysfunction and trigeminovascular pathways.
- Headaches from sinus disease are uncommon; most patients with "sinogenic pain" may actually have migraines or tension-type headaches.
- Imaging for acute rhinosinusitis is often not necessary, unless complications or concerns for serious causes, including facial swelling, orbital proptosis, and cranial nerve palsies.
- Sinus radiographs are often inaccurate; multiplanar computed tomography offers advantages of improved bony detail and can be done with low-dose protocols.
- MR imaging may be useful for complex sinus disease, distinguishing polyps, obstructive masses from inspissated secretions and fluid, infraorbital, or intracranial involvement.

INTRODUCTION

Rhinosinusitis is a common complaint present in 16% of the US population with annual economic burdens estimated at $22 billion.[1] Headaches are also extremely common, affecting 30% to 78% of the population, with US cost estimates of $100 million per million inhabitants per year.[2,3] These 2 conditions are among the top 10 reasons patients seek medical care, especially from otolaryngologists and neurologists.[4] Although patients and clinicians may self-diagnose their symptoms as a "sinus headache" or "rhinogenic headache," there is no true clinical definition for this entity.[5] Many studies have shown that so-called sinus headaches are in fact migraines in up to 88% to 90% of patients.[6,7] The Sinus, Allergy, and Migraine Study found that most patients self-diagnosing themselves or presenting to primary care physicians with a sinus headache from blockage or congestion were actually suffering from migraines.[8] Confounding the issue are the 2013

International Headache Society *International Classification of Headache Disorders* headache categories, which include 11.5 Headache attributed to disorder of the nose or paranasal sinuses, 11.5.1 Headache attributed to acute rhinosinusitis, and 11.5.2 Headache attributed to chronic or recurring rhinosinusitis (**Box 1**).[9] The similar overlapping symptoms of sinusitis and migraine likely occur due to similar anatomic autonomic, trigeminal nerve, vidian nerve, and the trigeminocardiac reflex pathways. This article reviews the anatomy, clinical cases, how imaging plays a role in assessment, and essential key clinical and radiographic findings that separate these entities.

NORMAL ANATOMY
Sinuses and Drainage Pathways

The air-filled spaces of the paranasal sinuses are lined with respiratory epithelium with cilia working together to clear secretions. At birth (**Fig. 1**), ethmoid and maxillary sinuses are present and

Disclosure Statement: Primal Pictures – Informa: Consultant.
Department of Radiology, Northwell Health, Zucker Hofstra School of Medicine at Northwell, North Shore University Hospital, 300 Community Drive, Manhasset, NY 11030, USA
* 171 East 84th Street Apt 26B, New York, NY 10028.
E-mail address: cfekirsch@gmail.com

Neuroimag Clin N Am 29 (2019) 227–241
https://doi.org/10.1016/j.nic.2019.01.003

Box 1
Classification of headache disorders

11.5. Headache attributed to disorder of the nose or paranasal sinuses. Previously used term: The term "sinus headache" is outmoded because it has been applied both to primary headaches and headache supposedly attributed to various conditions involving nasal or sinus structures. *Description:* Headache caused by a disorder of the nose and/or paranasal sinuses and associated with other symptoms and/or clinical signs of the disorder.

11.5.2. Headache attributed to chronic or recurring rhinosinusitis

Description: Headache caused by a chronic infectious or inflammatory disorder of the paranasal sinuses and associated with other symptoms and/or clinical signs of the disorder. Diagnostic criteria:

A. Any headache fulfilling criterion C

B. Clinical, nasal endoscopic, and/or imaging evidence of current or past infection or other inflammatory process within the paranasal sinuses

C. Evidence of causation demonstrated by at least 2 of the following:

   1. Headache has developed in temporal relation to the onset of chronic rhinosinusitis

   2. Headache waxes and wanes in parallel with the degree of sinus congestion, drainage, and other symptoms of chronic rhinosinusitis

   3. Headache is exacerbated by pressure applied over the paranasal sinuses

   4. In the case of a unilateral rhinosinusitis, headache is localized ipsilateral to it

D. Not better accounted for by another International Classification of Headache Disorders-3 (ICHD-3) diagnosis.

Comment: It has been controversial whether or not chronic sinus pathology can produce persistent headache. Recent studies seem to support such causation.

11.5.1. Headache attributed to acute rhinosinusitis

Description: Headache caused by acute rhinosinusitis and associated with other symptoms and/or clinical signs of this disorder.

Diagnostic criteria:

A. Any headache fulfilling criterion C

B. Clinical, nasal endoscopic, and/or imaging evidence of acute rhinosinusitis

C. Evidence of causation demonstrated by at least 2 of the following:

   1. Headache has developed in temporal relation to the onset of the rhinosinusitis

   2. Either or both of the following:

      a. Headache has significantly worsened in parallel with worsening of the rhinosinusitis

      b. Headache has significantly improved or resolved in parallel with improvement in or resolution of the rhinosinusitis

   3. Headache is exacerbated by pressure applied over the paranasal sinuses

   4. In the case of a unilateral rhinosinusitis, headache is localized ipsilateral to it

D. Not better accounted for by another ICHD-3 diagnosis.

Comments: 1. Migraine and 2. Tension-type headache can be mistaken for 11.5.1 Headache attributed to acute rhinosinusitis because of similarity in location and, in migraines, because of the commonly accompanying nasal autonomic symptoms. The presence or absence of purulent nasal discharge and/or other features diagnostic of acute rhinosinusitis help to differentiate. However, an episode of 1. Migraine may be triggered or exacerbated by nasal or sinus pathology. Pain as a result of pathology in the nasal mucosa or related structures is usually perceived as frontal or facial but may be referred more posteriorly. Finding pathologic changes on imaging of acute rhinosinusitis, correlating with the patient's pain description, is not enough to secure the diagnosis of 11.5.1 Headache attributed to acute rhinosinusitis. Treatment response to local anesthesia is compelling evidence, but may also not be pathognomonic.

From Headache Classification Committee of the International Headache Society (IHS). The International Classification of Headache Disorders, 3rd edition (beta version). Cephalalgia 2013;33(9):629–808.

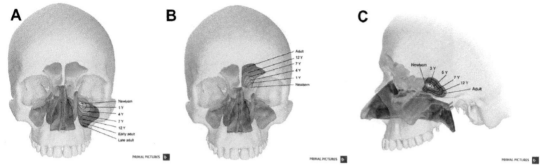

Fig. 1. (*A–C*) Sinus development. (*A, B*) Ethmoid and maxillary sinuses are present at birth and sites of infection in pediatric patients; the frontal sinuses arise from anterior ethmoidal air cells at around 6 years old. (*C*) Sphenoid sinus develops from age 2 years and pneumatizes at around age 8 years.

are the 2 major sites for infection in pediatric patients.[10] Sphenoid sinus pneumatization starts at about 9 months and the frontal sinuses at 7 to 8 years of age, with continuous expansion into adolescence. In children, acute rhinosinusitis (ARS) is a clinical diagnosis, and radiographic imaging is not indicated unless concerns for complications or surgical planning.[11] Imaging in patients with uncomplicated ARS is not proven to be useful, in that up to 80% of uncomplicated AR patients may have abnormal radiographic finding.[12]

Sinus anatomy is shown in **Fig. 2**. The superior frontal sinuses may be variable in size: 4% of the population may be hypoplastic and 5% to 8% of the population may be aplastic.[13,14] Frontal sinuses drain via the frontal recess, bordered by the fovea ethmoidalis, and the roof of the ethmoid air cells superiorly. At the anterior frontal recess margin is the agger nasi air cell, the most anterior ethmoid air cell. At the posterior frontal recess margin is the ethmoid bulla, located posterior superior to the hiatus semilunaris. The lateral wall of the olfactory fossa forms the medial frontal recess margin and the lamina papyracea the lateral margin; the opening of the frontal recess may vary depending on the attachment of the UP opening into either the infundibulum or the middle meatus.[15]

The nasolacrimal duct (NLD) (**Fig. 2**A) extends inferiorly from the ocular surface to the nasal cavity inferior meatus and contains an upper and lower canaliculus. The NLD walls are composed of helical connective tissue with a unique combination of microvilli, seromucous glands, lymphocytes, and macrophages[16] (**Fig. 2**A). An easy mnemonic to remember sinus drainage is anterior inferior–posterior superior. The most anterior structures, that is, the NLDs, drain to the inferior meatus; just behind them going posteriorly are the frontal recess, and anterior ostiomeatal complex draining the maxillary sinuses and anterior ethmoid air cells

into the middle meatus, the posterior ethmoid air cells, and the sphenoid sinus. The most posterior sinuses drain via the sphenoethmoidal recess into the superior meatus.

The ostiomeatal complex should be assessed for patency and is formed by the important bony uncinate process (UP) (**Fig. 2**B); this bone is what may be removed in functional endoscopic sinus surgery to visualize the maxillary sinus opening or ostium. Therefore, the radiologist and surgeon need to assess preoperatively that it is not attached or atelectatic to the orbital lamina papyracea.[17] The UP forms the medial maxillary infundibulum margin; the infundibulum is marked by pink arrows in **Fig. 2**B. The UP free edge superiorly forms the inferior hiatus semilunaris margin; this drains to the medial meatus and may vary anatomically, as in **Fig. 2**B, with a pneumatized uncinate tip.

SINUS ANATOMY: NEURAL AND VASCULATURE

Many neural pathways involving nociception, parasympathetic, and sympathetic nerves are involved with the paranasal sinuses. The nasal cavity takes inhaled air and filters, warms, humidifies the inhaled air, and is critical for perceiving noxious odors and stimuli. How smell works is yet to be completely elucidated, although CN I, the olfactory nerve, is critical, and CN V, the trigeminal nerve, also plays a role.

Cranial Nerve I: Olfactory Nerve

CN I, the unique olfactory nerve composed of unmyelinated axons with unique glia cells, has marked plasticity, allowing continual replacement of axons and remodeling in the central nervous system. However, CN I can also give viruses direct access intracranially. CN I joins axons forming fascicles "fila olfactoria," through the ethmoid lamina cribosa (cribriform plate

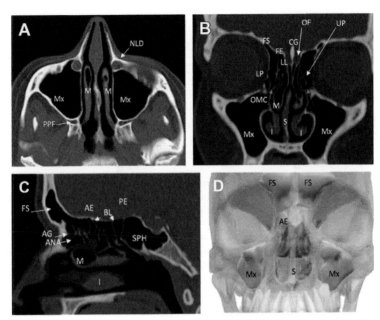

Fig. 2. (*A–D*) Bone window sinus CT normal paranasal sinuses axial plane (*A*), coronal plane (*B*), and sagittal plane (*C*). Sinus (*D*). AE, anterior ethmoid air cells, drain via ostiomeatal complex infundibulum to middle meatus, air space around middle turbinate; AG, Agger nasi (*Agger*, Latin for mound, pile, rampart; *Nasi*, nose), lateral nasal cavity ridge formed mucosa over maxilla ethmoidal crest; ANA, Agger nasi air cell, 90% of patients in lacrimal bone below AG, enlargement may obstruct frontal recess; BL, basal lamella (Latin *lamella*, small plate/flake), separates anterior and posterior ethmoid sinus, third basal lamella laterally attaches to lamina papyracea; CG, crista galli (Latin rooster crest) superior ethmoid bone above cribriform plate, attachment for anterior falx cerebri; FE, fovea ethmoidalis (Latin *fovea*, pit, depression) from the frontal bone forms ethmoid roof separating from anterior cranial fossa; FS, frontal sinus, drain frontonasal duct to anterior middle meatus; I, inferior turbinate (Latin turbinate inverted cone, scroll shaped, top), largest turbinate, deflects, humidifies, heats, filters air space or meatus; LL, lateral lamella, thinnest bone in the body, vertical lamella, joins inferior fovea ethmoidalis, variable height (Keros classification) affects olfactory fossa depth; LP, lamina papyracea (Latin *papyracea*, paper thin) from ethmoid bone, forms medial orbital wall, lateral ethmoid sinus; M, middle turbinate (also known as nasal concha, inferior ethmoidal turbinate, Latin *concha*, like seashell) when air filled, called concha bullosa; Mx, maxillary sinus, largest sinus drains to middle meatus; NLD, carries tears from eye to nasal cavity into inferior meatus; OF, olfactory fossa, contains olfactory nerve and bulb; OMC, ostiomeatal complex, pink arrows show the maxillary infundibulum, key drainage for the frontal, anterior ethmoid and maxillary sinuses, contains frontal recess, maxillary sinus ostium, ethmoidal infundibulum, hiatus semilunaris, middle meatus; PE, posterior ethmoid sinus, drains via sphenoethmoidal recess to the superior meatus with sphenoid sinus; S, nasal septum, separates nasal cavity formed by ethmoid perpendicular plate, vomer, crest of maxillary bone, crest of palatine bone, septal nasal cartilage, where the vomer and perpendicular plate of the ethmoid fuse there may be a bony spur; SPH, sphenoid sinus variable in shape, drains via sphenoethmoidal recess (or posterior ostiomeatal complex) to superior meatus; UP (Latin *uncinate*, hooked), note both of these are pneumatized, a normal anatomic variant. The UP arises from the lateral wall ethmoid cavity, a key component of the ostiomeatal complex, arises from ethmoid bone, superior edge forms an inferior margin of the hiatus semilunaris, and ethmoid bulla forms upper margin.

intracranially with sensory neurons connecting the brain and nasal cavity with no relay). The olfactory bulb circuitry contains olfactory axons and olfactory glomeruli.[18] Each olfactory bulb in the olfactory recess (Fig. 2B, Fig. 3), lateral to the crista galli, contains layered juxtaglomerular cells, containing periglomerular cells, external tufted cells, superficial short axon cells, mitral cells, and tufted cells. The olfactory pseudostratified columnar neuroepithelium has ciliated olfactory receptors in the nasal vault below the

cribriform plate and also extends to the superior nasal septum, superior turbinate, and superior lateral nasal wall in the olfactory cleft. There are 10 to 20 million cell bodies of primary olfactory receptor neurons.[19,20] These "filia olfactoria" nerves traverse the cribriform plate minute 15 to 20 openings and synapse in the olfactory bulb. The nasal cavity neuroepithelium along with olfactory receptor neurons contains microvillar cells, sustentacular cells, horizontal, globose basal cells, and Bowman gland duct

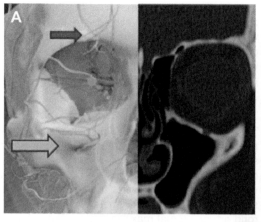
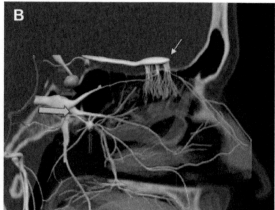
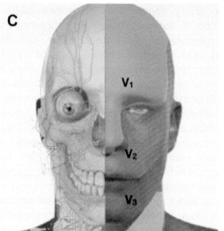
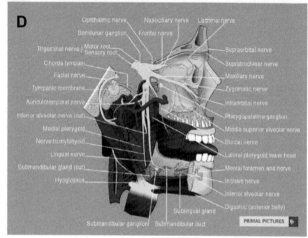

Fig. 3. (*A*) Coronal CT bone windows on the right side, with diagrammatic overlay on the left side showing the exit points of CN trigeminal branches. (*B*) Sagittal sinus CT with schematic overlay showing branches of CN I, olfactory nerve with filia olfactoria through the cribriform plate (*yellow arrow*), CN V branches including V$_1$, ophthalmic nerve that exits via the superior orbital fissure, with distal supraorbital branch (*small blue arrow*). V$_2$, maxillary nerve that exits via the foramen rotundum, synapses in the pterygopalatine ganglion (*red arrow*) to the infraorbital fissure and exits via the infraorbital foramen (*orange arrow*); and CN V$_3$, mandibular nerve (marked in green) that exits via the foramen ovale. (*C*) Sensory innervation distribution of the CN V trigeminal branches. (*D*) Detailed labeling in the sagittal plane of CN V trigeminal branches.

cells, which create mucus, allowing smell transduction.[21] Human olfactory neurons regenerate every 3 to 6 months, declining as one ages. Odor is detected by primary order olfactory receptors synapsing with second-order dendrites of mitral and tufted cells in the olfactory bulb glomerus and then is sent to anterior olfactory nucleus, olfactory tubercle, piriform cortex, lateral entorhinal cortex, amygdala cortical nucleus, periamygdaloid cortex, with fibers to the lateral hypothalamus and hippocampus, with smell intrinsically linked to memory.[22]

Cranial Nerve V: Trigeminal Nerve

The sensory supply of the paranasal sinuses is from V$_1$ ophthalmic and V$_2$ maxillary trigeminal

neural branches arising after the nerve exits intracranially via the superior orbital fissure, including as shown in **Fig. 3**.

CN V$_1$ ophthalmic nerve: exits intracranially via the superior orbital fissure, branches into 3 nerves: frontal, lacrimal, nasociliary.

> *Frontal nerve:* gives rise to the
> > Supraorbital nerve upper lid, frontalis muscle, scalp and branch to the frontal sinus
> > Supratrochlear nerve: supplies conjunctiva, upper lid forehead
> *Nasociliary nerve* gives rise to
> > *Posterior ethmoid nerve:* Arises before anterior ethmoid nerve, supplies posterior ethmoid and sphenoid sinus

Anterior ethmoid nerve: supplies frontal and anterior ethmoid sinus, anterior septum

Internal nerve: Lateral and medial branches

  External nasal nerve: supplies nasal tip skin

Infratrochlear nerve: arises near anterior ethmoidal foramen, runs along medial orbit, exits above medial canthus, supplies lateral nose above medial canthus, medial conjunctiva, and lacrimal apparatus.

Several long ciliary nerves enter glove with ciliary ganglion short ciliary nerves

Supplying cornea, iris, ciliary body, eye

CN V$_2$–Maxillary nerve: Exits via foramen rotundum to the pterygopalatine fossa and pterygopalatine ganglion and then continues via the inferior orbital fissure as the *infraorbital nerve* supplies sensory information midface, cheek, maxillary teeth.

Before foramen rotundum, a middle meningeal dural branch goes through foramen spinosum with the middle meningeal artery. After leaving the foramen rotundum, the nerve synapses in the pterygopalatine fossa give a zygomatic branch that divides to the zygomaticotemporal zygomaticofacial branches.

Anteriorly, the *infraorbital nerve* exits the infraorbital foramen and gives rise to the inferior palpebral, external and internal nasal branches, superior labial nerve medial and lateral branches.

Nasopalatine nerve via sphenopalatine foramen: goes incisive fossa hard palate

Superior alveolar nerves: anterior, middle, and posterior branches

Posterior superior nasal nerve: lateral branches superior and middle concha

Medical branches: nasal septum

Greater and lesser palatine nerves: branches perforate palatine bone perpendicular plate for sensation of mucosa over inferior nasal concha, inferior and middle meatus.[22–24]

Autonomic: Parasympathetic/Sympathetic Innervation

The general visceral efferent parasympathetic fibers arise from the superior salivatory nucleus and dorsal pontine lacrimal nucleus exiting into the cerebellopontine angle cistern via the nervus intermedius. The nervus intermedius exits via the internal auditory canal joining the facial nerve motor root and goes through the geniculate ganglion without synapsing to continue as the greater superficial petrosal nerve (GSPN).[25–28] The GSPN extends to the middle cranial fossa, picking up postganglionic sympathetic fibers from the internal carotid artery deep to the petrosal nerve and forms

the vidian nerve (also known as the nerve of the pterygoid canal). The vidian nerve exits via the vidian canal and synapses at the pterygopalatine ganglion with branches that subsequently innervate the minor salivary glands of the nasal cavity, palate, and paranasal sinuses.

Arterial Supply

The highly vascular nose is the only place where blood flows from lateral to medial; this means the arterial blood flow in the mucosa runs anteriorly opposite the direction of inspired air to warm it, with 3 major blood vessels. The key vessel is the sphenopalatine artery arising from the external carotid artery internal maxillary artery. The sphenopalatine artery divides into a septum internal artery and 2 external branches supplying the mucus membranes of the outer margin, concha, ethmoid, and sphenoid sinuses. Arterial supply also arises from the anterior and posterior ethmoid branches originating from the internal ophthalmic artery. Branches as in **Fig. 4**A, B with awareness and localization of the critical anterior and posterior ethmoid arteries are important to avoid inadvertent trauma to the vessels during functional endoscopic surgery. Vessels arising from the external carotid artery include, as noted above, the sphenopalatine artery, greater palatine, superior labial, and angular arteries. The nasal septum receives blood supply from the anterior and posterior ethmoid arteries superiorly and the sphenopalatine artery at the posterior inferior margin, the greater palatine posteriorly, and the labial artery anteriorly. These terminal vessels converge at the inferior anterior third region of the nasal septum, also known as "Little area" after Dr Little, a portion of the septum at risk for nose bleeds, with a highly vascular supply at the transition point between respiratory and squamous epithelium known as "Kiesslbach plexus," essentially a 1.5-mm^2 area of capillary loops; bleeding from either anterior or posterior vessels can result in nosebleeds (epistaxis), one of the most common ear, nose, and throat (ENT) emergencies.

Venous Drainage

The nasal venous supply lacks valves (**Fig. 4**C, D) and accompanies arterial vessels perforating the maxillary bone from the facial, maxillary, infraorbital, and palatine arteries. The veins drain into the anterior facial vein and with venous plexuses at the interior nasal conchae, inferior meatus, and nasal septum posteriorly into a pterygoid plexus. Veins from the orbital ophthalmic plexus join with ethmoidal veins. Venous drainage can vary going either intracranially, intraorbitally, or both. Upper

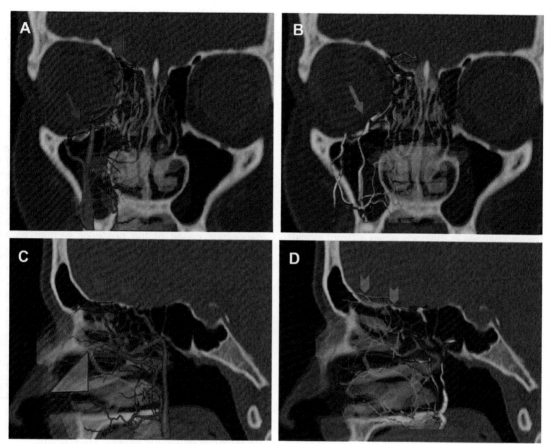

Fig. 4. (A–D) Bone window sinus CT with arterial supply (A) coronal, (B) sagittal and venous drainage, (C) coronal, (D) sagittal. (A, B) Sphenopalatine artery divides internal artery of the septum external branches (*red arrow*) anterior and posterior ethmoid branches (*red chevrons*) from ICA ophthalmic artery. The nasal septum anterior and posterior ethmoid arteries superiorly and sphenopalatine artery, greater palatine posteriorly, and labial artery anteriorly converge at the inferior anterior third region of the nasal septum. Little triangle in light yellow shows terminal vessels and region at risk for epistaxis. Venous drainage (C, D), veins follow along arterial pathways and venous drainage may either go to the pterygoid plexus, facial vein, along the orbit or intracranially to the superior sagittal sinus, cavernous, or sphenoparietal sinus.

nasal cavity and frontal sinus veins drain into the interior calvarium via cribriform plate foramina and foramen cecum to the superior longitudinal sinus, superior sagittal sinus, or sphenoparietal sinus.[29] Importantly, pathogens spreading via the veins from the sinuses through the lamina papyracea may be why rhinosinusitis is the predominant cause of pediatric orbital infections.[30–33] The direct connection of veins along the frontal lobes at the orbital margin, via cribriform plate and foramen cecum to the superior sagittal sinus, also allows infections to spread via this route intracranially with risk for venous sinus thrombosis.

Trigeminocardic Reflex

The blood flow of nasal vessels running opposite to inspired air is controlled via autonomic reflexes.

The trigeminal nerve ophthalmic V_1 and maxillary V_2 have afferent fibers sending the sensation of the paranasal sinuses to the trigeminal brainstem sensory nuclear complex, which includes the spinal trigeminal nucleus, thalamus, and somatosensory cortex. Autonomic sympathetic stimulation is from nerve fibers arising from the superior cervical ganglion via the deep petrosal nerve branch of the vidian nerve; these fibers join with parasympathetic fibers from the CN VII superior salivatory nucleus that form the GSPN. Together the deep petrosal nerve and GSPN form the vidian nerve synapsing in the sphenopalatine ganglion. Both the trigeminal nerve endings and the parasympathetic nerves end in the basal cells of the nasal epithelium.[34] Sympathetic stimulation in the nasal cavity decreases blood flow and in doing so decongests the nasal venous erectile tissue.[29,35]

Pain in the nasal cavity occurs via the Ad fast responding mechanoreceptor pain fibers and slower unmyelinated C fibers. Activated fibers release tachykinins, including substance P, neurokinin A, and neuropeptide K.[34] Sympathetic stimulation is associated with neuropeptide Y, along with norepinephrine, and parasympathetic fibers cause release of acetylcholine and vasoactive intestinal peptide.[25,34,36,37].

Because the chemicals and neurotransmitters for paranasal nerve activation are the same as those found in migrainelike headaches, rhinogenic pain and allergic rhinitis often mimic each other, and therein is the conundrum.[34,38–40] Stimulation of the paranasal trigeminal nerves may cause reflexive changes in the body when afferent signals go to the trigeminal medullary sensory nucleus, where internuncial neurons in the reticular formation link to efferent parasympathetic vagus neurons in the motor nucleus with resultant vagal symptoms, including cardiac bradyarrhythmia, gastric hypermotility, and hypotension.[41] Although most "rhinogenic headaches" are migraines, approximately 80% to 90% of the time, there are cases where paranasal sinus pathologic condition can be responsible for headaches, as illustrated in the following set of clinical cases.

Clinical Cases

Sphenoid sinusitis

Sphenoid sinusitis is a unique entity seen in approximately 3% of all sinusitis cases, which if delayed or misdiagnosed can result in high morbidity and mortality.[10,42–44] Headache is often the most common symptom in sphenoid sinusitis, and clinical and endoscopic assessment may be limited for assessment of disease. Because only a thin bony margin separates the sphenoid sinus from adjacent meninges, cavernous sinus, including the internal carotid arteries, cranial nerves III, IV, V, and VI, clivus, and pons, these structures are at risk in patients with severe sphenoid sinus disease. Patients with sphenoid sinusitis can present with headache, worse on standing, bending, movement, or coughing, with periorbital pain, and greater than 50% of patients may have a fever.[10,42,45] Unfortunately, physical examination is limited, and this diagnosis is often delayed; a key clue is the presence of a continuous increasing headache, CN V pain and paresthesia, photophobia, and eye tearing, with the headache causing sleep interference not relieved by analgesics.[10,42] Concern for sphenoid sinus pathologic condition requires imaging as seen in **Fig. 5A–I**, either via computed tomography (CT) or MR imaging, and if concern for vascular involvement as

demonstrated in this case, additional imaging, including CT angiography and interventional cerebral angiogram, may be warranted. These cases may result in complex pathology and require collaborative skills of otolaryngology and neurosurgery.[44]

Epistaxis

Although epistaxis and migraine headaches may occur together, the exact causes are not well elucidated; however, as noted above, epistaxis is one of the most common ENT emergencies and may occur along the anterior nasal septum from involvement of Little or Kisselbach plexus. Severe dangerous cases of the posterior septum may result in airway compromise.[46] Tumors within the nasal fossa may present with nonspecific findings, which can lead to a delay in diagnosis; therefore, clinicians should pay special attention to clinical signs of nasal obstruction with epistaxis because these signs are suggestive of an underlying mass[47] (**Fig. 6**). Tumoral masses in the paranasal region, like all cancers in the head and neck, should prompt a careful radiographic assessment of the pterygopalatine fossa and ganglion, for loss of the fat planes, enlargement and enhancement of trigeminal and facial branches, including the vidian GSPN and deep petrosal nerves to evaluate for potential perineural tumoral involvement.[26]

In young male patients with epistaxis, nasal obstruction, and headache, a juvenile nasopharyngeal angiofibroma needs to be excluded.[48] These rare highly vascular tumors typically involve male adolescents and may also track along the skull base foramina intraorbitally or intracranially, as in **Fig. 7**.

Benign lesions may also obstruct the nasal cavities; interestingly, obstruction in and of itself may not necessarily cause pain or headache because the sinuses may be insensitive to pain.[10,49] The pain experienced in the sinus region may be a reflection of autonomic system engorgement with inflamed nasal structures along the nasofrontal ducts, turbinates, ostia, and upper nasal areas. True sinus headaches are reported to be more of a dull deep aching quality, with heaviness and fullness that does not present with nausea or vomiting.[10,49] The last important clinical case of epistaxis, shown in **Fig. 8**, is of an inverting papilloma or Schneiderian papilloma inverted type.

These locally aggressive benign lesions may recur and can be associated with carcinoma.[50] These are usually in male patients 50 to 70 years of age, with tumor arising from the lateral nasal wall of the ostiomeatal complex of the middle meatus often involving the maxillary sinus, with

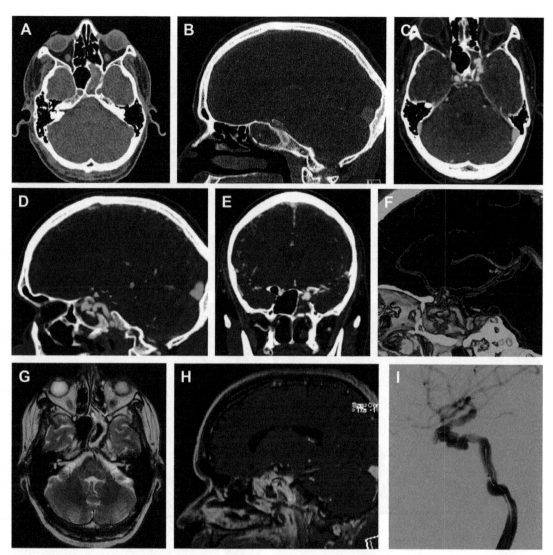

Fig. 5. (*A*) CT scan of the paranasal sinuses in the (*A*) axial plane, (*B*) sagittal plane of a geriatric female patient transferred from a nursing home, with a history of diabetes complaining of headache, demonstrating a left sphenoid sinus mucocele with foci of increased attenuation likely inspissated secretions or fungal infection in patient with aspergillus infection and dehiscence left lateral sphenoid bony margin, concerning for cavernous sinus and carotid artery involvement. (*C–F*) CT angiogram (*C*) axial plane, (*D*) sagittal plane, (*E*) coronal plane, and (*F*) 3-dimensional CT angiogram reconstruction showing multilobulated pseudoaneurysm of the left internal cavernous carotid artery. (*G*) Axial T2 MR imaging. Note lack of T2 signal in the left sphenoid sinus, from inspissated secretions with lack of mobile free water hydrogens making the sinus appear dark and aerated compared with (*H*) sagittal T1 postcontrast MR imaging demonstrating the enhancing mucosal margins, opacified left sphenoid mucocele, and multilobulated left internal carotid artery pseudoaneurysm projecting into the left sphenoid sinus. (*I*) Cerebral angiography of the left internal cavernous carotid artery multilobulated pseudoaneurysm with catheter in situ. The pseudoaneurysm and left cavernous ICA were coiled, and the patient had good collateral flow to the left middle cerebral artery via patient anterior and posterior communicating arteries.

unilateral nasal obstruction and epistaxis as the most common presenting symptoms. Causes are unknown; however, research has suggested that human papillomavirus (HPV) may be associated. HPV is a well-established cause for oropharyngeal carcinoma; of note, the sinonasal cavity is emerging as an additional critical area for transcriptionally active HPV-related tumors, a factor that should be taken into consideration when evaluating patients with recurrent nasal obstruction and headache with or without epistaxis.[51–54]

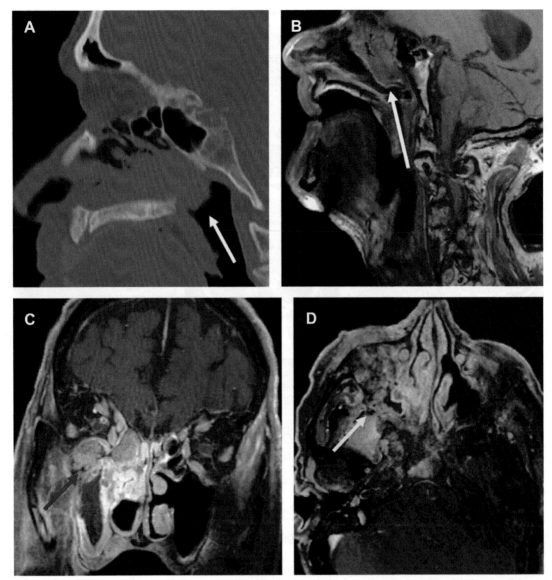

Fig. 6. (*A*) Sagittal CT, (*B*) sagittal T1 MR imaging in an 83-year-old man with nasal obstruction and epistaxis, and tumoral mass obstructing the right nasal cavity (*white arrows*), determined to be squamous cell carcinoma. Patient underwent surgical resection and radiation. (*C, D*) Coronal and axial T1 postcontrast gadolinium MR imaging with fat saturation, obtained 6 months later; patient with recurrent nasal obstruction, tumor, posterior epistaxis, and headache. (*C*) Perineural involvement (*red arrow*) along the right V₂ maxillary nerve in the infraorbital foramen lifting the right inferior rectus muscle superiorly. (*D*) Involvement of the right pterygopalatine fossa and pterygomaxillary fissure (*yellow arrow*). Perineural tumor involvement was also noted on the vidian nerve (GSPN) and right geniculate ganglion.

How to Image

Computed tomography

CT is a primary modality of choice for imaging the paranasal sinuses and assessment of the bony architecture and osseous margins. However, like all ionizing radiation imaging modalities, care must be taken to reduce unnecessary radiation exposure to radiosensitive organs, including the thyroid gland or orbit. CT imaging may be acquired using noncontrast, high-resolution, thin-section axial images reconstructed in the coronal and sagittal plane using both soft tissue and bone window algorithms. Contrast may be given in cases whereby there is concern for complications, including subperiosteal abscess, epidural or subdural empyema, osteomyelitis, tumor,

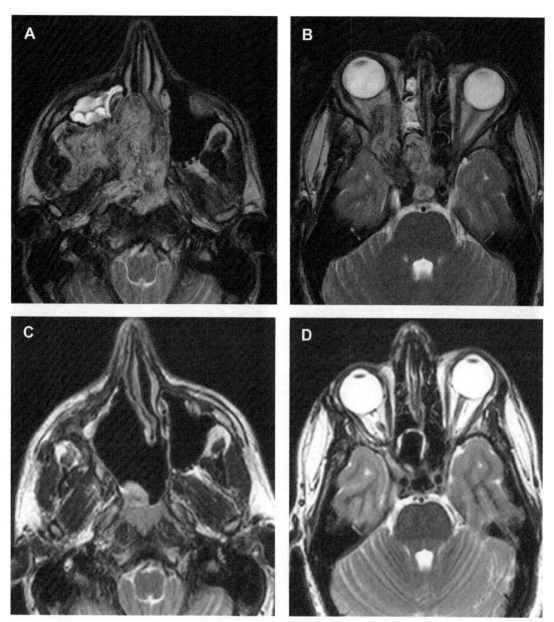

Fig. 7. (*A, B*) Axial T2 in a 17-year-old man with nasal obstruction and epistaxis, with hypervascular mass widening the pterygopalatine fossa, displacing the posterior maxillary sinus margin anteriorly with intraorbital and intracranial extension and right orbital exophthalmos. Patient underwent embolization via cerebral angiography and surgical resection. (*C, D*) Posttreatment axial T2, in the same planes, with removal of the mass, median antrectomy, turbinectomy and septectomy, and postoperative right orbital enophthalmos.

venous thrombosis, or concern for vessel involvement with additional imaging, including CT angiography or venography, as shown in **Fig. 5.** Iodinated contrast is used for contrast in CT; because of its increased electron density and higher atomic number ($Z = 53$), it has a radiodensity of approximately 25 to 30 HU/mg mL with tube voltages of 100 to 120 kVp.[1,15,55–58]

MR imaging

MR imaging offers a better assessment of soft tissue characteristics, extent of tumor, and/or infectious or inflammatory processes, including perineural spread, as seen in **Fig. 6,** and for assessing intraorbital or intracranial extension. Sequences used include high-resolution (3 mm) T1- and T2-weighted images of the sinonasal cavities with inclusion of the orbit, skull base, and

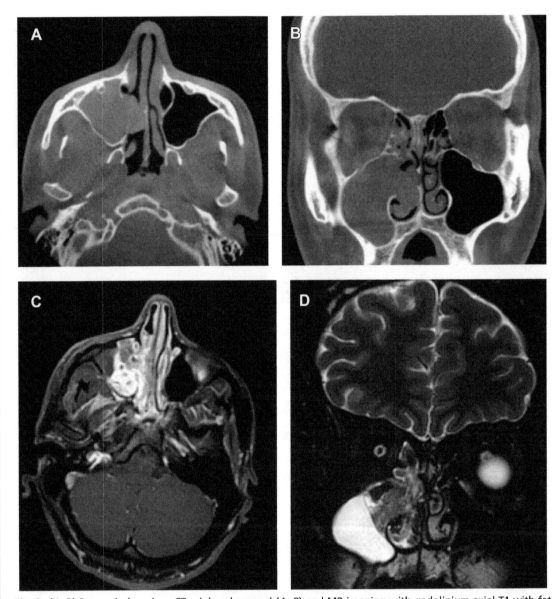

Fig. 8. (*A–D*) Bone window sinus CT axial and coronal (*A, B*) and MR imaging with gadolinium axial T1 with fat saturation (*C*) and coronal short TI inversion recovery (STIR) MR imaging (*D*), with a right inverting papilloma obstructing the right ostiomeatal complex with right maxillary mucocele. (*D*) The coronal MR imaging STIR sequence is able to separate the soft tissue component from the trapped bright secretions seen laterally, as opposed to the corresponding coronal sinus CT in (*B*).

adjacent intracranial regions; gadolinium contrast, which is paramagnetic because of 7 unpaired electrons, may be used. This shortens T1 and causes areas of increased vascularity or extravasation, as seen in **Figs. 5–7**, to appear bright on T1-weighted sequences.[1,15,57,58]

Essential Clinical Findings

Although updated criteria for rhinosinusitis still include "pain" as an indicator for sinusitis, research has shown a poor correlation between facial pain and headache and sinus disease, with many cases of self-diagnosed or referred "rhinosinusitis" actually being migraines.[5–8,59,60] Current diagnostic criteria for chronic rhinosinusitis include 12 weeks of nasal obstruction, congestion, anterior/posterior nasal discharge, facial pain/fullness, and decreased sense of smell, with objective verification of mucosal inflammation, polyps, or purulent discharge via CT or nasal endoscopy.[59,60] In fact, when headache and facial pain are eliminated as one of the symptom-based criteria for chronic rhinosinusitis, the specificity of clinically and radiographically diagnosed sinusitis improves.[59,60] However, not all "rhinogenic headaches" are always migraines; in patients with a dull ache or epistaxis, or patients at risk for complications from sinusitis, imaging is vital for assessment of involvement of deep tissue planes, intraorbital or intracranial extension.

SUMMARY

Headaches and sinus disease are common complaints with overlapping symptoms secondary to the autonomic innervation, with a marked worldwide prevalence. Most self-diagnosed "rhinogenic headaches" are actually migraines. However, certain headaches can signal sinus pathologic condition, and clinical history is important, especially in patients with dull, unrelenting positional headaches that may signal sphenoid sinus involvement. Awareness of the critical bony, vascular, and neural anatomy, clinical symptoms, and clinical history is vital. In patients with obstruction, nasal epistaxis, severe infectious or inflammatory pathologic condition, imaging is critical to assess vascular, orbital, or intracranial involvement, and treatment may require coordinated team involvement of Radiology, Otolaryngology, Neurology, and Neurosurgery.

REFERENCES

1. Kirsch CFE, Bykowski J, Aulino JM, et al. ACR appropriateness criteria® sinonasal disease. expert panel on neurologic imaging. J Am Coll Radiol 2017; 14(11S):S550–9.
2. Cashman EC, Smyth D. Primary headache syndromes and sinus headache: an approach to diagnosis and management [review]. Auris Nasus Larynx 2012;39(3):257–60.
3. Jensen R, Rasmussen BK. Burden of headache. Expert Rev Pharmacoecon Outcomes Res 2004; 4(3):353–9.
4. St Sauver JL, Warner DO, Yawn BP, et al. Why patients visit their doctors: assessing the most prevalent conditions in a defined American population. Mayo Clin Proc 2013;88(1):56–67.
5. Gryglas A. Allergic rhinitis and chronic daily headaches: is there a link? [review]. Curr Neurol Neurosci Rep 2016;16(4):33.
6. Schreiber CP, Hutchinson S, Webster CJ, et al. Prevalence of migraine in patients with a history of self-reported or physician-diagnosed "sinus" headache. Arch Intern Med 2004;164(16):1769–72.
7. Cady RK, Schreiber CP. Sinus headache: a clinical conundrum [review]. Otolaryngol Clin North Am 2004;37(2):267–88.
8. Eross E, Dodick D, Eross M. The Sinus, Allergy and Migraine Study (SAMS). Headache 2007;47(2): 213–24.
9. Headache Classification Committee of the International Headache Society (IHS). The International Classification of Headache Disorders, 3rd edition (beta version). Cephalalgia 2013;33(9): 629–808.
10. Marmura MJ, Silberstein SD. Headaches caused by nasal and paranasal sinus disease [review]. Neurol Clin 2014;32(2):507–23.
11. Magit A. Pediatric rhinosinusitis [review]. Otolaryngol Clin North Am 2014;47(5):733–46.
12. Gwaltney JM Jr, Phillips CD, Miller RD, et al. Computed tomographic study of the common cold. N Engl J Med 1994;330(1):25–30.
13. Earwaker J. Anatomic variants in sinonasal CT. Radiographics 1993;13:381–415.
14. Lee WT, Kuhn FA, Citardi MJ. 3D computed tomographic analysis of frontal recess anatomy in patients without frontal sinusitis. Otolaryngol Head Neck Surg 2004;131:164–73.
15. Mossa-Basha M, Blitz AM. Imaging of the paranasal sinuses [review]. Semin Roentgenol 2013;48(1): 14–34.
16. Paulsen F. The human nasolacrimal ducts [review]. Adv Anat Embryol Cell Biol 2003;170. III–XI, 1–106.
17. Beale TJ, Madani G, Morley SJ. Imaging of the paranasal sinuses and nasal cavity: normal anatomy and clinically relevant anatomical variants. Semin Ultrasound CT MR 2009;30:2–16.
18. Crespo C, Liberia T, Blasco-Ibáñez JM, et al. Cranial pair i: the olfactory nerve. Anat Rec (Hoboken) 2018. https://doi.org/10.1002/ar.23816.
19. Tavakoli A, Schmaltz A, Schwarz D, et al. Quantitative association of anatomical and functional classes of olfactory bulb neurons. J Neurosci 2018;38(33): 7204–20.
20. Hadley K, Orlandi RR, Fong KJ. Basic anatomy and physiology of the olfaction and taste. Otolaryngol Clin North Am 2004;37:1115–26.
21. Leopold DA, Hummel T, Schwob JE, et al. Anterior distribution of the human olfactory epithelium. Laryngoscope 2000;110:417–21.
22. Wrobel BB, Leopold DA. Olfactory and sensory attributes of the nose. Otolaryngol Clin North Am 2005; 38(6):1163–70.
23. Prendergast PM. Neurologic anatomy of the nose. In: Shiffman M, Di Giuseppe A, editors. Advanced aesthetic rhinoplasty. Berlin: Springer; 2013.
24. Hu KS, Kwak HH, Song WC, et al. Branching patterns of the infraorbital nerve and topography within the infraorbital space. J Craniofac Surg 2006;17(6): 1111–5.

25. Baraniuk JN. Sensory, parasympathetic, and sympathetic neural influences in the nasal mucosa [review]. J Allergy Clin Immunol 1992;90(6 Pt 2): 1045–50.

26. Kirsch CFE, Schmalfuss IM. Practical tips for MR Imaging of perineural tumorspread [review]. Magn Reson Imaging Clin N Am 2018;26(1):85–100.

27. Brackmann DE, Fetterman BL. Cranial nerve VII: facial nerve. In: Goetz GC, editor. Textbook of clinical neurology. Philadelphia: Saunders Elsevier; 2007. p. 185–98.

28. McClurg SW, Carrau R. Endoscopic management of posterior epistaxis: a review [review]. Acta Otorhinolaryngol Ital 2014;34(1):1–8.

29. Van Cauwenberge P, Sys L, De Belder T, et al. Anatomy and physiology of the nose and the paranasal sinuses [review]. Immunol Allergy Clin North Am 2004;24(1):1–17.

30. Chandler JR, Langenbrunner DJ, Stevens ER. The pathogenesis of orbital complications in acute sinusitis. Laryngoscope 1970;80(9):1414–28.

31. Kirsch CFE. Orbital infection. eMedicine; 2015. Available at: https://emedicine.medscape.com/article/383902-overview#showall.

32. Sciarretta V, Demattè M, Farneti P, et al. Management of orbital cellulitis and subperiosteal orbital abscess in pediatric patients: a ten-year review. Int J Pediatr Otorhinolaryngol 2017;96:72–6.

33. Sanchez TG, Cahali MB, Murakami, et al. Septic thrombosis of orbital vessels due to cutaneous nasal infection. Am J Rhinol 1997;11(6):429–33.

34. Mehle ME. What do we know about rhinogenic headache? The otolaryngologist's challenge [review]. Otolaryngol Clin North Am 2014;47(2): 255–64.

35. Jones N. The nose and paranasal sinuses physiology and anatomy [review]. Adv Drug Deliv Rev 2001;51(1–3):5–19.

36. Sessle BJ. Acute and chronic craniofacial pain: brainstem mechanisms of nociceptive transmission and neuroplasticity, and their clinical correlates. Crit Rev Oral Biol Med 2000;11:57–91.

37. Baraniuk JN. Neurogenic mechanisms in rhinosinusitis. Curr Allergy Asthma Rep 2001;1:252–61.

38. Mehle ME. Migraine and allergy: a review and clinical update. Curr Allergy Asthma Rep 2012;12(3):240–5.

39. Bellamy J, Cady R, Durham P. Salivary levels of CGRP and VIP in rhinosinusitis and migraine patients. Headache 2006;46:24–33.

40. Gelfand EW. Inflammatory mediators in allergic rhinitis. J Allergy Clin Immunol 2004;114:S135–8.

41. Chowdhury T, Mendelowith D, Golanov E, et al. Trigeminocardiac reflex: the current clinical and physiological knowledge. J Neurosurg Anesthesiol 2015; 27(2):136–47.

42. Nour YA, Al-Madani A, El-Daly A, et al. Isolated sphenoid sinus pathology: spectrum of diagnostic and treatment modalities. Auris Nasus Larynx 2008;35(4):500–8.

43. Friedman A, Batra PS, Fakhri S, et al. Isolated sphenoid sinus disease: etiology and management. Otolaryngol Head Neck Surg 2005;133(4):544–50.

44. Braun JJ, Debry C, Imperiale A, et al. Imaging sphenoid diseases. Clin Radiol 2018. https://doi.org/10.1016/j.crad.2018.03.006.

45. Deans JA, Welch AR. Acute isolated sphenoid sinusitis: a disease with complications. J Laryngol Otol 1991;105(12):1072–4.

46. Ranieri A, Topa A, Cavaliere M, et al. Recurrent epistaxis following stabbing headache responsive to acetazolamide. Neurol Sci 2014;35(Suppl 1): 181–3.

47. Kharoubi S. Malignant tumor's of nasal fossae: anatomoclinic's study and a new classification: study about 21 cases. Cancer Radiother 2005;9(3): 187–95 [in French].

48. Tang IP, Shashinder S, Gopala Krishnan G, et al. Juvenile nasopharyngeal angiofibroma in a tertiary centre: ten-year experience. Singapore Med J 2009;50(3):261–4.

49. Wolff HG. Wolff's headache and other facial pain. 1st edition. New York: Oxford University Press; 1948.

50. Prado FA, Weber R, Romano FR, et al. Evaluation of inverted papilloma and squamous cell carcinoma by nasal contact endoscopy. Am J Rhinol Allergy 2010; 24(3):210–4.

51. Wood JW, Casiano RR. Inverted papillomas and benign nonneoplastic lesions of the nasal cavity [review]. Am J Rhinol Allergy 2012;26(2): 157–63.

52. Adelstein DJ, Ridge JA, Gillison ML, et al. Head and neck squamous cell cancer and the human papillomavirus: summary of a National Cancer Institute State of the Science Meeting, November 9–10, 2008, Washington, DC. Head Neck 2009;31(11): 1393–422.

53. Lewis JS Jr, Westra WH, Thompson LD, et al. The sinonasal tract: another potential "hot spot" for carcinomas with transcriptionally-active human papillomavirus [review]. Head Neck Pathol 2014; 8(3):241–9.

54. Kamalian S, Lev MH, Gupta R. Computed tomography imaging and angiography -principles. Handb Clin Neurol 2016;135:3–20.

55. Bulla S, Blanke P, Hassepass F, et al. Reducing the radiation dose for low-dose CT of the paranasal sinuses using iterative reconstruction: feasibility and image quality. Eur J Radiol 2012;81(9):2246–50.

56. Lusic H, Grinstaff MW. X-ray-computed tomography contrast agents. Chem Rev 2013;113(3): 1641–66.

57. Fatterpekar GM, Delman BN, Som PM. Imaging the paranasal sinuses: where we are and where we are going. Anat Rec (Hoboken) 2008;291(11):1564–72.

58. Bricker A, Stultz T. Imaging for headache: what the neuroradiologist looks for. Otolaryngol Clin North Am 2014;47(2):197–219.

59. Levine HL, Setzen M, Cady RK, et al. An otolaryngology, neurology, allergy, and primary care consensus on diagnosis and treatment of sinus headache. Otolaryngol Head Neck Surg 2006; 134(3):516–23.

60. Hirsch SD, Reiter ER, DiNardo LJ, et al. Elimination of pain improves specificity of clinical diagnostic criteria for adult chronic rhinosinusitis. Laryngoscope 2017;127(5):1011–6.

Headache in Chiari Malformation

Abraham F. Bezuidenhout, MD[a], Yu-Ming Chang, MD, PhD[a], Carl B. Heilman, MD[b],
Rafeeque A. Bhadelia, MD[c],*

KEYWORDS

- Chiari malformation • Chiari 1 malformation • Headache • Cough-associated headache

KEY POINTS

- The majority of Chiari I malformation (CMI) patients experience headaches, but not all such headaches can be directly attributable to the diagnosis.
- Transient cough-associated headache is the most distinctive symptom of CMI.
- Certain routine imaging findings may suggest that the headache in a CMI patient is likely associated with the diagnosis, but their absence does not preclude an association.
- A normal cine phase-contrast study suggests that the headache is not caused by CMI. However, an abnormal cerebrospinal fluid (CSF) flow study is only moderately predictive of an association between the headache and CMI.
- Real-time CSF flow imaging with coughing as a physiologic challenge holds great promise for an objective evaluation of CMI patients with headache, but further studies are needed.

 Video content accompanies this article at http://www.neuroimaging.theclinics.com.

INTRODUCTION

Chiari malformations are a collection of hindbrain and craniocervical junction abnormalities (Table 1), of which Chiari I malformation (CMI) is the most commonly seen type in clinical practice, with a reported prevalence of 0.56% to 0.75% on MRI.[1,2] The main imaging feature of CMI is cerebellar tonsillar herniation of 5 mm or greater below the level of foramen magnum (Fig. 1),[3] with headache being the most common symptom.[4] Recently, many have questioned this anatomic criteria for the diagnosis of CMI given that many fitting this criteria are asymptomatic or have no specific symptoms related to tonsillar herniation.[5] Nevertheless, until a better criterion emerges, the degree of tonsillar herniation has remained the only accepted definition of CMI. Many patients with primary or congenital CMI are believed to have a skull base bony abnormality,[6] which can vary from a shallow posterior fossa, retroflexed odontoid, or short basilar process, to fusion between the occiput and C1. The term secondary or acquired CMI is often used when tonsillar herniation meeting the diagnostic criteria for CMI is caused by downward pressure by a posterior fossa mass or results from intracranial hypotension or intracranial hypertension.[6] For the purpose of this discussion, CMI will be used to refer to primary or congenital CMI, and when referring to secondary or acquired CMI, it will be specifically stated.

Disclosure Statement: Nothing to disclose.
[a] Department of Radiology, Beth Israel Deaconess Medical Center, 1 Deaconess Road, Boston, MA 02215, USA;
[b] Department of Neurosurgery, Tufts Medical Center, 800 Washington Street, Boston, MA 021152, USA;
[c] Department of Radiology, Harvard Medical School, Beth Israel Deaconess Medical Center, 1 Deaconess Road, Boston, MA 02215, USA
* Corresponding author.
E-mail address: rbhadeli@bidmc.harvard.edu

Neuroimag Clin N Am 29 (2019) 243–253
https://doi.org/10.1016/j.nic.2019.01.005

Table 1
Types of chiari malformations

Type of Chiari Malformation	Pathology and Imaging Findings
Chiari I • Chiari 0 • Chiari 1.5	5-mm ≥ Cerebellar tonsillar herniation below foramen magnum Small posterior fossa and syringomyelia without tonsillar herniation below foramen magnum Cerebellar tonsillar plus obex herniation below foramen magnum
Chiari II	Herniation of cerebellum and hindbrain below foramen magnum plus lumbar myelomeningocele
Chiari III	Cranio-cervical meningo-encephalocele
Chiari IV	Cerebellar hypoplasia

Chiari II, III, and IV usually present with severe neurologic abnormalities in the neonatal period or early childhood,[7] and headache is typically not a presenting or important symptom. Given the preponderance of data available related to headache in CMI regarding types of headache,

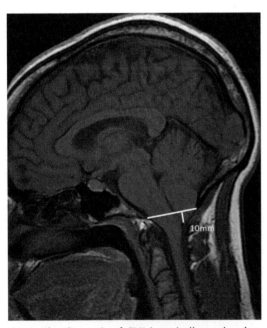

Fig. 1. The diagnosis of CMI is typically made when there is 5 mm or greater downward displacement of the cerebellar tonsils below the foramen magnum as measured on sagittal MRI. In this patient, a 10 mm tonsillar herniation is seen.

pathophysiology, and imaging features, discussion of headache in this article will be limited to CMI.

TYPES AND LOCATION OF HEADACHE IN CHIARI I MALFORMATION

Prevalence of headache of any type in CMI is believed to be around 81% of patients at presentation.[8] The headaches experienced by CMI patients are transient activity-associated (related to activities such as coughing, Valsalva, sneezing, laughing, or exercise, but are collectively known as cough-associated), migraine, tension-type, or of the cluster variety.[9] Of all headache types experienced by CMI patients, transient cough-associated (seconds to <5 min duration) is the most distinctive and is seen in approximately one-third of patients.[9,10] In a study of 30 CMI patients, the authors found 9 patients (30%) presented with typical cough-associated headache.[11] Recently, Curone and colleagues[10] found that 87% of CMI patients with headache complained of some increase in intensity with cough or other activities. However, only 34% of their patients had short-lasting cough-associated headache. Thus, it is essential to distinguish the change in intensity of long-lasting headaches with cough or other activities from typical cough-associated headaches of CMI by their temporal relationship and short duration. The criteria for the diagnosis for headache attributed to CMI has been established by the International Headache Society (IHS), and it is important for a radiologist interpreting CMI imaging studies to be aware of these criteria to aid in clinical decision making (Box 1).[12]

Although CMI headaches are characteristically cough-associated, they need to be differentiated from primary cough headache.[13,14] In clinical practice, cough-associated headaches are reported by about 1% of patients getting consultation for headaches.[15] It is reported that nearly two-thirds of patients with cough-associated headache have an MRI-demonstrable abnormality in the posterior fossa, and 90% of them have CMI.[9] The remaining one-third of headaches is classified as primary or benign cough headache. The major clinical distinction between primary and secondary cough-associated headache is that the primary cough-associated headaches are generally seen in older patients (>60-year in age).[9] They are characterized by bilateral posterior headaches that are temporally related to cough and last for a few seconds to minutes but can last up to 2 hours, show a male preponderance, and respond well to treatment with pain medications.[15]

As opposed to primary cough-headache, the secondary cough-associated headaches are seen in younger (<40 years of age) patients; they are predominantly sub-occipital and have female preponderance. In a recent study by Alperin and colleagues,[16] 85% of patients with cough-associated headache and CMI were female. Given the high prevalence of posterior fossa abnormalities in young patients with cough-associated headache, it is recommended that all these patients should undergo an MRI examination to exclude a posterior fossa abnormality such as CMI.[9] In addition to the brief episodes of cough-associated headaches, many CMI patients can have continuous or long-lasting headaches.[17] Some CMI patients can also have continuous daily headache (CDH) and in some, CDH can be exaggerated by cough. A hypothetical relationship between CDH and CMI has been suggested but not proven by controlled clinical studies.[9]

IHS defines Chiari attributed cough-associated headache to be typically suboccipital in location. However, many variations of that pattern exist. These variations are in their association with cough and also in their location. For example, some CMI patients have brief cough-associated headaches that are not suboccipital but could be frontal or on the side of head. Alperin and colleagues[18] divided CMI-associated headaches in 3 categories. In 63 CMI patients with headache, 40 patients (63%) had suboccipital Valsalva-related headaches; 15 patients (24%) had suboccipital headache not related to Valsalva, and 8 patients (13%) had nonoccipital non-Valsalva-related headaches (it should be noted that the terms cough- and Valsalva-related headache are often used interchangeably). For the authors' ongoing research endeavors in CMI patients with headache, different classifications and location of headaches have been determined, as demonstrated in **Table 2**.

Table 2
Authors' proposed classification of headaches in Chiari I malformation

Type of Headache	Characteristics of Headache
Type 1	• Transient localized suboccipital cough-related headaches (headache triggered by cough, Valsalva, sneezing, exercise, bending forward, or laughing)
Type 2	• Transient localized nonoccipital or generalized cough-related headaches
Type 3	• Constant localized (occipital or nonoccipital) or generalized headache (constant daily headache) that may be exacerbated by cough
Type 4	• Transient or constant suboccipital headaches that are not cough related
Type 5	• Transient or constant localized nonoccipital or generalized headaches that are not cough related

PATHOPHYSIOLOGY OF HEADACHE IN CHIARI MALFORMATION

It is generally agreed that the underlying pathophysiology of cough-associated headache in CMI is the result of impaired CSF flow between the head and spine secondary to tonsillar herniation and neural crowding at the foramen magnum.[19] However, consensus has not been reached as to how the CSF flow obstruction produces cough-associated headache.

Previously published invasive pressure studies by Williams and Sansur and colleagues described pressure changes in the head and spine in CMI patients with cough-associated headache.

Williams assessed pressure changes at rest and after coughing in CMI patients and showed that physiologic challenges such as coughing or Valsalva maneuver produce pressure dissociation between the head and spine.[20] The development of pressure dissociation is explained by an initial elevation of spinal pressure (from increased intrathoracic pressure and consequent distension of the epidural veins) during coughing, displacing CSF to the head (Fig. 2). However, immediately after coughing, this displaced CSF returns with relative ease to the spinal canal in a healthy patient but not in a patient with CMI because of impaction of the cerebellar tonsils, thereby creating a pressure dissociation between the head and spine, where intracranial pressure is higher than that of the spine (see Fig. 2B, D). The transiently increased intracranial pressure results in a brief headache by stimulation of pressure receptors of the dura. It was also shown by Williams that there was minimal to no pressure dissociation in these CMI patients at baseline or rest (in absence of cough).

Sansur and colleagues[21] measured spinal intrathecal pressures and observed increased pressures at baseline and during coughing in patients with CMI and cough-associated headache compared with CMI patients without cough-associated headache and normal subjects. They suggested that headache in CMI may be caused by the absolute value of spinal CSF pressure reached during a cough and concluded that elevated spinal CSF pressure in CMI patients with cough-associated headache is associated with significant foramen magnum obstruction to CSF flow, which increases intracranial pressure and results in the headache.

IMAGING APPROACH AND IMAGING FINDINGS
Anatomic Imaging

It is the authors' experience that in most patients with CMI, diagnosis is usually made on a routine brain or cervical spine MRI obtained to evaluate headache, neck pain, and paresthesia or for other unrelated reasons such as trauma evaluation. The diagnosis of CMI is made when there is 5 mm or greater downward displacement of the cerebellar tonsils below the foramen magnum (see Fig. 1). Tonsillar displacement of 3 to 5 mm is often referred to as tonsillar ectopia, and less than 3 mm tonsillar herniation is considered to be within normal limits.[3] From here, the imaging approach depends on what information is already available and the clinical circumstances of the initial imaging. The main goal for any additional imaging is to assess the brain, spinal cord, and the craniocervical junction.

Brain
Routine brain imaging is required to exclude hydrocephalus, mass, or manifestations of intracranial hypotension, often referred to as acquired CMI. Use of gadolinium is warranted when a posterior fossa mass is suspected, which can displace the cerebellar tonsils downwards and mimic primary CMI. Gadolinium is also useful when intracranial hypotension is suspected (such as with positional headache elicited in the upright position that is relieved when lying down), which is characterized in imaging by diffuse pachymeningeal enhancement.

Spinal cord
In patients with CMI, imaging of the entire spinal cord is required to exclude a spinal cord syrinx (syringohydromyelia). A syrinx is seen in up to 34% to 40% of patients with CMI.[2,22,23] Syrinx is generally defined as linear/cylindrical CSF intensity collection in the spinal cord of 2 mm or greater width.[22] A linear CSF collection in the central aspect of the spinal cord less than 2-mm is generally considered a prominent central canal. In patients with an unequivocal diagnosis of CMI, the authors do not recommend use of gadolinium for evaluation of spinal cord syrinx. However, many recommend the use of contrast at the initial evaluation but not for the follow-up. Many CMI patients with syrinx also complain of headache, but the exact number has not been previously reported.

Cranio-cervical junction imaging
The authors use high-resolution 3-dimensional T2-weighted images like FIESTA or CISS for dedicated imaging of the craniocervical junction. These images provide exquisite detail of CSF spaces in the region and help assess some of the findings that will be described.

Anatomic imaging is generally considered to be less reliable in predicting which patients have CMI-associated headache.[11,18] However,

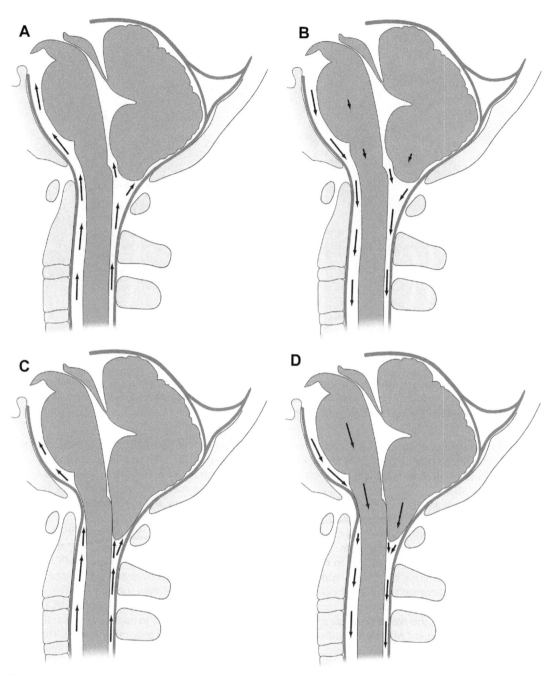

Fig. 2. (*A, B*) Control patient; (*C, D*) CMI patient. During coughing there is an elevation of spinal pressure (from increased intrathoracic pressure and consequent distension of the epidural veins), which displaces CSF to the head (*A, C*). However, immediately after coughing, this displaced CSF returns with relative ease to the spinal canal in a healthy patient (*B*), but not in a patient with CMI because of further impaction of the cerebellar tonsils. This creates pressure dissociation between the head and spine, where intracranial pressure is higher than spinal pressure (*D*).

there are certain anatomic imaging findings that suggest the patient's headache may be related to CMI. Degree of tonsillar decent of greater than 12 mm, deformity of the tonsils with a pointed shape, crowding of the neural structures, and

effacement of the retro-cerebellar cisterns are findings that suggest that the headache is more likely to be associated with CMI[2] (**Fig. 3**A). In contrast, tonsillar herniation without obliteration of fourth ventricular recess and rounded tonsils

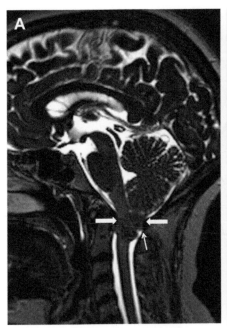
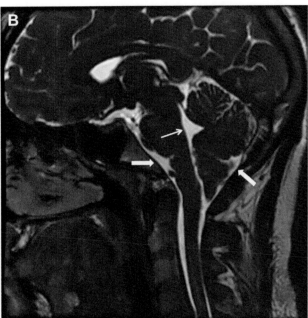

Fig. 3. (A) Anatomic imaging findings suggesting the patient's headache symptoms are related to CMI include tonsillar herniation of 14 mm (>12 mm), pointed shape of the tonsils (skinny arrow), crowding of the neural structures, and effacement of the retrocerebellar cisterns (block arrows). (B) Anatomic imaging findings suggesting that headache symptoms are likely not associated with CMI include tonsillar herniation of 10 mm (<12 mm) without obliteration of fourth ventricular recess (skinny arrow) and rounded tonsils with open subarachnoid space at the cervicomedullary junction/foramen magnum (block arrows).

with open subarachnoid space at the cervicomedullary junction/foramen magnum are less likely to be suggestive of the headache associated with CMI (Fig. 3B).

Milhorat and colleagues[8] also measured dimensions of the posterior cranial fossa with MRI and suggested that in CMI patients with cough-associated headache, the posterior fossa is smaller than those without it, leading to reduced compliance and therefore headache from transiently elevated intracranial pressure. Alperin and colleagues[18] (2015) measured several anatomic and physiologic (CSF and blood flow) parameters and demonstrated that in CMI patients with cough associated suboccipital headache, intracranial volume (and thereby compliance) is lower than those without cough-associated suboccipital headache.

Physiologic Imaging

Although anatomic MRI provides detailed information about foramen magnum narrowing through assessment of the degree of tonsillar herniation and crowding of the neural structures, these findings are poorly correlated with the type and severity of headaches experienced by CMI patients.[11,18] Because it is generally agreed that CMI-associated headache is caused by impairment of

CSF flow at the level of the foramen magnum, motion-sensitive MRI techniques (mainly cine phase-contrast [cine-PC]) have been used to help guide patient management. Cine-PC is available on most scanners and can be utilized in patients with CMI. Sagittal cine-PC provides an excellent means for qualitative visual inspection of CSF spaces at the craniocervical junction, and the authors use them extensively. Axial cine-PC is important for quantitative evaluation of velocity profile and calculation of flow rates.[24–26] The authors generally use a velocity encoding (VENC) of 5 to 7 cm/s with a superior to inferior directional encoding in scanning adult patients with CMI. The VENC can be increased to 10 to 15 cm/s in children to eliminate the potential for velocity aliasing. Quantitative evaluation requires dedicated software for analysis. Hofkes and colleagues[27] used sagittal and axial cine-PC to correlate different CSF flow patterns with CMI symptomatology. The authors use sagittal qualitative assessment of cine-PC to grade severity of CSF flow obstruction in CMI (Fig. 4, Table 3, Videos 1–4).

Work correlating CSF flow abnormalities at the cranio-cervical junction with CMI patient head type and anatomic abnormalities at the foramen magnum has been performed by McGirt and colleagues,[28] used cine-PC imaging in 33 patients

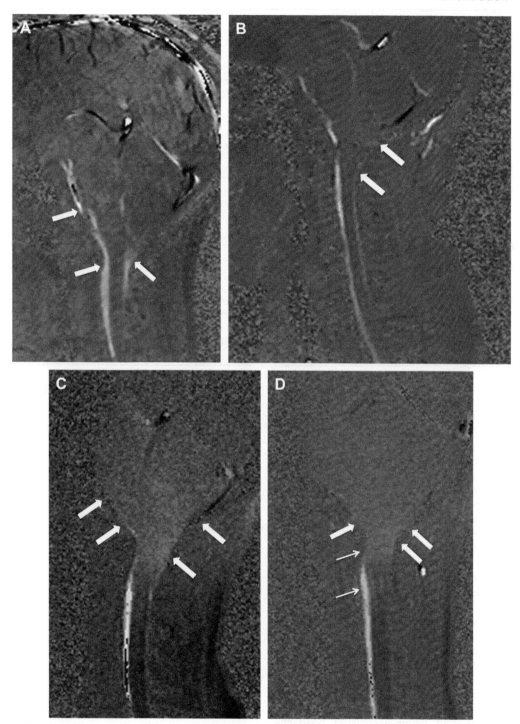

Fig. 4. (*A–D*) Different severities (qualitative) of craniocervical junction CSF flow obstruction on cine-PC images in a patient with CMI. (*A*) Demonstrates a normal CSF flow pattern as evidenced by continuous uninterrupted anterior CSF systolic flow with flow also noted in the posterior fossa as well as posterior to the upper cervical cord (*block arrows;* CSF diastolic phase not shown). (*B*) Demonstrates mild obstruction as evidenced by normal anterior flow, but decreased/absent flow in the posterior fossa and posterior to the upper cervical cord (*block arrows*). (C) Demonstrates moderate obstruction as evidenced by partially interrupted anterior systolic flow at the level of the foramen magnum as well as absent flow in the posterior fossa and posterior to the upper cervical cord (*block arrows*). (*D*) Demonstrates severe obstruction as evidenced by interrupted CSF systolic flow at the foramen magnum (*block arrow*), asynchronous flow between the level just below the foramen magnum and the C2-C4 level (*skinny arrow*), as well as absent flow in the posterior fossa and posterior to the upper cervical cord (*block arrows*).

Table 3
Qualitative interpretation of craniocervical junction cerebrospinal fluid flow on cine-phase contest images in patient with Chiari I malformation

CSF Flow Pattern	Anterior CSF Flow	Posterior CSF Flow
Normal (see Fig. 4A, Video 1)	• Continuous uninterrupted bidirectional systolic and diastolic flow present • Flow immediately below foramen magnum is synchronous with flow at C2-3 and C3-4	• Foramen Magendie/fourth ventricular flow present • Posterior upper cervical flow present
Mild obstruction (see Fig. 4B, Video 2)	• Normal	• Foramen Magendie/4th ventricular flow: decreased or absent • Posterior to upper cervical cord (below tonsils) flow decreased but present
Moderate obstruction (see Fig. 4C, Video 3)	• Partially interrupted bidirectional systolic and diastolic flow (flow interruption seen in a couple to several phase)	• Foramen Magendie/4th ventricular flow absent. • Posterior to upper cord (below tonsils) flow absent
Severe obstruction (see Fig. 4D, Video 4)	• Interrupted bidirectional systolic and diastolic flow at foramen magnum • Flow immediately below foramen magnum asynchronous with flow at C2-3 and C3-4	• Foramen Magendie/fourth ventricular flow absent • Posterior to upper cord (below tonsils) flow absent

with CMI. In this study, CSF flow abnormalities on cine-PC were defined as absence of normal biphasic CSF flow within any of the aqueduct, fourth ventricle, foramen of Magendie, foramen magnum, around the cerebellar tonsils, prepontine cistern, and ventral or dorsal to the upper cervical spinal cord. Headaches were divided in to frontal/generalized or occipital. They observed that CMI patients with frontal and generalized headache were 10 times less likely to demonstrate CSF flow abnormalities at the craniocervical junction and 8 times less likely to have tonsillar herniation greater than 7 mm compared with CMI patients with occipital headache. The most important conclusion of this study was that a frontal or generalized headache in the setting of normal cine-PC study (see Fig. 4A) indicates that the headache is not related to CMI and will not benefit from surgery.

Bhadelia and colleagues[11] (2011) studied 30 CMI patients with cine-PC and evaluated differences in the CSF flow pattern between CMI patients with and without cough-related headache. Nine of the 30 patients had cough-associated headache, which was defined as short-lasting occipital headache initiated or aggravated by cough, exertion, or a Valsalva-like maneuver. It was observed that in CMI patients with cough-associated headache, prolonged CSF diastolic flow duration was seen compared to those without cough-associated headache. This can be seen by observing the presence of persistent CSF diastolic flow below foramen magnum on cine-PC images (Fig. 5).

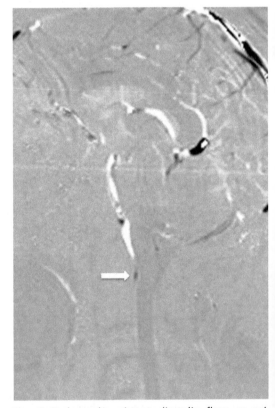

Fig. 5. Prolonged/persistent diastolic flow as evidenced by black signal (*block arrow*) just below the foramen magnum compared with systolic flow (white signal) at other levels above and below which more frequently seen in CMI patients with cough-associated headaches.

By assessing CSF and blood flow with cine-PC, Alperin measured cardiac cycle-related intracranial volume changes, intracranial compliance, and MRI-derived intracranial pressure.[18] The results indicated that CMI patients with cough-associated suboccipital headache had lower intracranial volume change, lower intracranial compliance index, and higher MRI-derived intracranial pressure compared with CMI patients with other types of headaches.

Bhadelia and colleagues evaluated cough-associated changes in CSF flow by utilizing a novel real-time pencil-beam MRI technique.[19] Those interested in the detailed description of the technique are referred to previous publications.[19,29] Each real-time scan was acquired for approximately 90 seconds, during which time the patient was asked to: breathe quietly for the first 15 to 20 seconds, then cough as forcefully as possible consecutively 6 times, and breathe quietly again after the end of coughing period until the end of the acquisition time. Results provided the first objective demonstration of CSF flow changes in CMI patients with cough-associated headache.[19,29] In CMI patients with cough-associated headache, a brief 10- to 15-second decrease in CSF flow was observed below the foramen magnum (Fig. 6A). However, such a decrease in CSF flow after coughing was not observed in CMI patients without typical transient cough-associated headache (Fig. 6B). These findings are thus congruent with Williams' initial proposal of the underlying pathophysiology of cough headache in CMI patients, which hypothesized that there is decreased CSF flow after coughing below foramen magnum (see Fig. 2).[20]

PEARLS AND PITFALLS

Transient cough-associated headaches are the most distinctive symptom of Chiari I malformation. It is important to assess CSF pathways at the craniocervical junction with high-resolution T2-weighted images as well as with cine-PC to help in the management of a CMI patient with headache. Conditions such as intracranial hypotension need to be excluded before making a diagnosis of CMI.

WHAT THE REFERRING PHYSICIAN NEEDS TO KNOW

It is not sufficient for the radiologist to simply describe the extent of cerebellar tonsil herniation in CMI. In order to provide imaging information that may be used by the clinician to determine if a patient's headache is likely attributable to CMI, the report should include

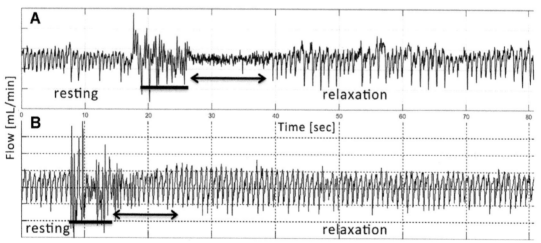

Fig. 6. Real-time MRI in 2 different CMI patients with headache demonstrating the effect of coughing on cardiac cycle–related CSF flow waveforms. The x-axis indicates time in seconds; the y-axis, CSF flow rate in milliliters per minute. Left-to-right: resting, coughing (*underlined*), after coughing (*underlined with double-headed arrows*), and relaxation waveforms are seen. CSF stroke volume is the average of the absolute flow from craniocaudal and caudocranial CSF flow. (A) (*upper panel*) From a 39-year-old CMI female patient with transient cough-associated headache lasting for about 10 to 15 seconds. Immediately after coughing, there is more than 50% decrease in CSF flow seen lasting for about 12 seconds (*underlined with double headed arrows*), which then returns to normal during the relaxation period (compare resting and relaxation phases with postcoughing phase). (B) (*lower panel* From a 34-year old female CMI patient with continuous daily headache. No decrease in CSF flow is seen after coughing, which remains at similar magnitude as resting and relaxation phases (compare resting and relaxation phases with postcoughing phase).

- Whether the tonsils are deformed and pointed versus in a rounded configuration
- If there is obliteration of the retrocerebellar CSF space and foramen of Magendie
- If the CSF pathways of the anterior and posterior cervicomedullary junction are patent or obliterated
- If cine-PC imaging is available, then CSF flow along these pathways should be assessed and described as normal or obstructed (mild, moderate, or severe)
- If there are bony abnormalities such as basilar invagination, retroflexed odontoid, or craniocervical fusion.
- If a syrinx is visualized, evaluation of the entire spinal cord should be recommended
- If brain imaging has not been performed, this should be recommended to exclude secondary causes of tonsillar herniation

SUMMARY

Headache is a common symptom in patients with CMI, characterized by 5 mm or greater cerebellar tonsillar herniation below foramen magnum. It is important for the radiologist to be aware of the different types of headaches reported by a CMI patient and which headache patterns are distinctive features of the diagnosis. A methodical imaging strategy is required to fully assess a CMI patient to exclude secondary causes of tonsillar herniation such as intracranial hypotension or associated conditions such as syrinx. Both anatomic and physiologic imaging can help determine if headaches are CMI associated, and assist clinicians in therapeutic decision making.

SUPPLEMENTARY DATA

Supplementary data related to this article can be found online at https://doi.org/10.1016/j.nic.2019.01.005.

REFERENCES

1. Meadows J, Kraut M, Guarnieri M, et al. Asymptomatic Chiari type I malformations identified on magnetic resonance imaging. J Neurosurg 2000;92:920–6.
2. Elster AD, Chen MY. Chiari I malformations: clinical and radiologic reappraisal. Radiology 1992;83:347–53.
3. Aboulezz AO, Sartor K, Geyer CA, et al. Position of cerebellar tonsils in the normal population and in patients with Chiari malformation: a quantitative approach to MR imaging. J Comput Assist Tomogr 1985;9:1033–6.
4. Voelker R. Chiari conundrum: researchers tackle a brain puzzle for the 21st century. JAMA 2009;301:147–9.
5. Baisden J. Controversies in Chiari I malformations. Surg Neurol Int 2012;3:S232–7.
6. Mehta A, Chilakamarri P, Zubair A, et al. Chiari headache. Curr Pain Headache Rep 2018;22:49.
7. Hadley DM. The Chiari malformations. J Neurol Neurosurg Psychiatry 2002;72(Suppl 2):ii38–40.
8. Milhorat TH, Chou MW, Trinidad EM, et al. Chiari I malformation redefined: clinical and radiographic findings for 364 symptomatic patients. Neurosurgery 1999;44:1005–17.
9. Riveira C, Pascual J. Is Chiari type I malformation a reason for chronic daily headache. Curr Pain Headache Rep 2007;11(1):53–5.
10. Curone M, Valentini LG, Vetrano I, et al. Chiari malformation type 1-related headache: the importance of a multidisciplinary study. Neurol Sci 2017;38(Suppl 1):91–3.
11. Bhadelia RA, Frederick E, Patz S, et al. Cough-associated headache in patients with Chiari I malformation: CSF flow analysis by means of cine phase-contrast MR imaging. AJNR AM J Neuroradiol 2011;32:739–42.
12. The International classification of headache disorders 3rd edition. Available at: https://www.ichd-3.org/7-headache-attributed-to-non-vascular-intracranial-disorder/7-7-headache-attributed-to-chiari-malformation-type-i-cm1/. Accessed July 26, 2016.
13. Pascual J. Primary cough headache. Curr Pain Headache Rep 2005;9:272–6.
14. Headache Classification Subcommittee of the International Headache Society. The international classification of headache disorders. Cephalalgia 2004;24(Suppl 1):8–160.
15. Pascual J, González-Mandly A, Berciano J, et al. Cough headache: our experience in the MRI era. Headache 2005;45:775–6.
16. Alperin N, Sivaramakrishnan A, Lichtor T. Magnetic resonance imaging-based measurements of cerebrospinal fluid and blood flow as indicators of intracranial compliance in patients with Chiari malformation. J Neurosurg 2005;103:46–52.
17. Stovner LJ. Headache associated with Chairi type I malformation. Headache 1993;33:175–81.
18. Alperin N, Loftus JR, Oliu CJ, et al. Imaging-based features of headaches in Chiari malformation type I. Neurosurgery 2015;77:96–103.
19. Bhadelia RA, Patz S, Heilman C, et al. Cough-associated changes in CSF flow in Chiari I malformation evaluated by real-time MRI. AJNR Am J Neuroradiol 2016;37:825–30.
20. Williams B. Cough headache due to craniospinal pressure dissociation. Arch Neurol 1980;37:226–30.
21. Sansur CA, Heiss JD, De Vroom HL, et al. Pathophysiology of headache associated with cough in

patients with Chiari I malformation. J Neurosurg 2003;98:453–8.

22. Gad KA, Yousem DM. Syringohydromyelia in patients with Chiari I malformation: a retrospective analysis. AJNR Am J Neuroradiol 2017;38:1833–8.

23. Strahle J, Muraszko KM, Garton HJL, et al. Syrinx location and size according to etiology: identification of Chiari-associated syrinx. J Neurosurg Pediatr 2015;16:21–9.

24. Quigley MF, Iskandar B, Quigley ME, et al. Cerebrospinal fluid flow in foramen magnum: temporal and spatial patterns at MR imaging in volunteers and in patients with Chiari I malformation. Radiology 2004;232:229–36.

25. Haughton V, Mardal KA. Spinal fluid biomechanics and imaging: an update for neuroradiologists. AJNR Am J Neuroradiol 2014;35:1864–9.

26. Bhadelia RA, Bogdan AR, Kaplan RF, et al. Cerebrospinal fluid pulsation amplitude and its quantitative relationship to cerebral blood flow pulsations: a phase-contrast MR flow imaging study. Neuroradiology 1997;39:258–64.

27. Hofkes SK, Iskandar BJ, Turski PA, et al. Differentiation between symptomatic Chiari I malformation and asymptomatic tonsillar ectopia by using cerebrospinal fluid flow imaging: initial estimate of imaging accuracy. Radiology 2007;245: 532–40.

28. McGirt MJ, Nimjee SM, Floyd J, et al. Correlation of cerebrospinal fluid flow dynamics and headache in Chiari I malformation. Neurosurgery 2005;56: 716–21 [discussion: 716–21].

29. Bezuidenhout AF, Khatami D, Heilman CB, et al. Relationship between cough-associated changes in CSF flow and disease severity in Chiari I malformation: an exploratory study using real-time MRI. AJNR Am J Neuroradiol 2018;39: 1267–72.

Headache and Aneurysm

O-Ki Kwon, MD, PhD

KEYWORDS

- Aneurysm • Headache • Pathophysiology • Trigeminal nerves • Upper spinal nerves

KEY POINTS

- No pain from the aneurysm develops without pain nerves.
- The pain nerves involved in headache are the trigeminal nerve and high cervical spinal nerves (C1, 2, and 3).
- The pain nerves for intradural structures are present on blood vessel (mainly artery) walls.
- Various types of stimulation to the arterial walls producing pain include compression, distension, traction, chemicals, and simple touching.
- With the basic knowledge, the mechanism of the headache from cerebral aneurysms can be better understood.

INTRODUCTION

Headache requires a wider definition than just a pain in the head.[1,2] In this article, a narrow concept of headache (a pain) is used. It is a basic concept that headache develops from peripheral pain nerve fibers. No headache develops without pain nerves. Brain does not have pain nerve fibers.[3] Therefore, as seen in awake brain surgery, direct surgical manipulation of the brain does not produce pain. Structures that have pain fibers are dura (pachymeninges), major arteries, and veins. The entire dura does not sense pain. Pain is perceived only in dural parts with pain nerve fibers. Likewise, the other source of intracranial pain-cerebral vessels can also produce pain only when they have pain fibers.

CONTENT

Nerves that innervate intracranial vessels are autonomic (sympathetic and parasympathetic) and sensory nerves. Direct innervation from fibers of the brain may be present[4] but its function is not yet fully determined. The pain nerves involved in headache are trigeminal nerve (and its 3 divisions) and high cervical spinal nerves (dorsal [sensory] roots of C1, 2, and 3). The sensory trigeminal nerve

fibers terminate in caudal and interpolar divisions of the spinal trigeminal nucleus. The sensory fibers of cervical spinal nerves terminate in the dorsal horns of the spinal cord. Small fibers of the general somatic afferent system of cranial nerve VII (through parts of the nervus intermedius), IX (tympanic nerve, nerve of Jacobson), and X (auricular nerve, Arnold nerve) also have nociception but the sensing area is limited to ear structures. The cell bodies that receive these pain senses are also in the trigeminal nucleus. The central nervous system itself contributes to relation, perception, and modulation of the headache. Centrally produced pain such as thalamic pain, in which no activation of peripheral nerve fibers is necessary for generating pain, exists but it is not a typical form of headache. The brain stem itself may also have headache-producing structures,[5,6] but it is not thought to be a mainstay mechanism of headache development. Stimulation or modulation of the trigeminal nucleus and its connections may be a pain-producing mechanism in this situation.

The exact mechanisms that cause major primary headaches like migraines, tension headaches, and cluster headaches are still not clearly understood. Proposed theories are divided into peripheral origin (arteries and accompanying trigeminal or cervical spinal nerves) and central

Department of Neurosurgery, Seoul National University Bundang Hospital, Gumiro 173 Beongil, Bundanggu, Seongnamsi, Gyeonggido 463-707, South Korea
E-mail address: meurokwonoki@gmail.com

Neuroimag Clin N Am 29 (2019) 255–260
https://doi.org/10.1016/j.nic.2019.01.004
1052-5149/19/© 2019 Elsevier Inc. All rights reserved.

(brain) origin. Unlike primary headaches, the headache associated with aneurysms has a definite peripheral origin, the aneurysm. In general, cerebral aneurysms arise from major cerebral arteries on which pain nerve fibers are present. These nerves are branches from the trigeminal nerve (almost all from V1, the ophthalmic division) and the upper 3 cervical spinal nerves.

All of the 3 trigeminal divisions have sensory nerves. Their main sensing structures are dura. The ophthalmic division of the trigeminal nerve (V1) innervates the anterior cranial fossa and falx through the anterior and posterior ethmoidal nerves. The tentorial nerve is the first branch of the ophthalmic nerve. It takes a recurrent course to innervate the superior surface of the tentorium and posterior falx. The maxillary nerve (V2) innervates part of the dura of the anterior and middle cranial fossa. The mandibular nerve (V3) also innervates part of the anterior and middle cranial fossa dura.

In general, these nerves use vessels (mainly arteries) to reach dura (via meningeal arteries) and intracranial structures (via internal carotid artery). Sympathetic nerves also use a similar pathway.

Supratentorial intradural structures are innervated mainly by branches of V1. It enters the intradural space along with the ICA. It begins from cavernous sinus and dura around the ICA level. On the surface of the ICA, the fibers go along into the middle cerebral artery (MCA) and anterior cerebral artery (ACA) as with the ICA course. The exact level at which they end seems to vary.

Posterior cranial fossa dura and intradural structures, mainly arteries, are innervated by C1, C2, and C3. The cervical spinal nerve 1 (C1) is unique. Unlike other spinal nerves that have both motor and sensory fibers, only about half of C1 has sensory fibers.[7] It enters the skull with the hypoglossal nerve.

How far and how many these pain nerves reach on the dura seem to vary. Distribution of pain sense is not uniform over the dura. A study of awake brain surgery showed that the intensity of pain differed by location. The intensity of the pain caused by touching the temporal part of the skull base dura was 7.9 out of 10 (range, 0–10), falx and tentorium was 4.2 (range, 0–9), and perisylvian leptomeninges was 6.6 (range, 0–10).[8] Convexity dura has less pain. Stimulation of some parts of the dura does not induce pain. Likewise, large areas of posterior fossa dura over rostral and lateral convexities of the cerebellum were insensitive to pain by stimulation.[9]

The proximal portions of arteries have more abundant sensory innervation than distal. Proximal arterial segments near the circle of Willis were exquisitely sensitive to stimuli but were progressively less sensitive over the convexity.[10,11] In awake brain surgery, neurosurgeons confirmed that pain-sensitive structures are the dura of the skull base, falx cerebri, and the leptomeninges of the sylvian fissure and neighboring sulci.[9] Some sensory fibers reach opercular or proximal cortical segments of MCA.

Several types of stimulation on cerebral arteries produce pain, including dilatation (distension), traction, chemical, thermal, and electrical stimulation.[10–12] Among these, dilation of intracranial and extracranial arteries has been studied extensively.[12,13] Balloon inflation of cerebral arteries caused headaches, which disappeared immediately with balloon deflation.[12] Stent-assisted coiling caused headache more than simple coiling.[14,15]

Simpler manipulation like just touching of the arteries can also produce pain. Experience from awake brain surgery has provided information about pain-sensitive structures.[8] In most cases, just touching causes pain. The pain from these structures was described as sharp, acute, intense, and brief. When the touching stopped, the pain disappeared. The pain from large aneurysms or tumors could be explained by just touching (compression with low pressure) of neighboring pain-sensitive structures.

Displacement of the ICA also produces pain.[16] Frequent development of frontal and periorbital pain after stent-assisted coiling of ICA aneurysms can be explained by ICA stretching and displacement.[17]

As with other sensory neurons, activation of pain fibers is influenced by temporal and spatial summation. The number of nociceptive receptors and neurons can be related with pain strength.[18,19] Low-intensity stimulation for a short duration may not produce pain. Likewise, slowly forming aneurysms may not induce headache. Acute tearing dissection[20] or acute formation of a daughter sac or a pseudoaneurysm from a pre-existing aneurysm could produce sudden severe headache. This headache may disappear if there is no further acute change or it may persist if other subsequent arterial changes, such as rupture, that newly stimulate pain nerve fibers on the arterial wall occur.

In addition, neural adaptation could affect pain production and its intensity, so the intensity of pain caused by long-lasting low-grade stimulation may decrease over time despite pain sensation, especially via C-type nociceptive fibers, adapts slowly. New headaches can develop after coiling or stent-assisted coiling, probably caused by stretching of arterial walls, and generally are of low intensity and spontaneously disappeared days or weeks later.[14,15]

Patients have pulsatile or throbbing headache with increased intracranial pressure. Increased pulsatility of the whole dura can be a mechanism for headache. Increased arterial pulsatility can also contribute to headache.[21-23] Likewise, the pulsatile motion of aneurysms may be a source of headache. Conditions with high pulsatile movement, such as large size and thin wall, may be factors of headache development. The pulsatile motion can be reduced or removed by treatment. Disappearance of headache after coil packing of aneurysmal sacs can be explained by this mechanism.[21] Many reports have showed that headache had substantial reductions after treatment, including surgery and coiling.[24-29]

Acute severe stimulation, such as abrupt arterial tearing or distension of major cerebral arteries, causes a sudden intense headache such as thunderclap headache. Vasospasm, also produces severe pain from the uncontrollable smooth muscle contraction and compensatory dilatation. The same one can be the mechanisms of pain associated with reversible cerebral vasoconstriction syndrome (RCVS).

Long-lasting stimulation with constant intensity could have diverse results. Pain fiber activation may decrease with adaptation, or, in some situations, temporal summation can provoke more severe headache. Prolonged intensive headache from subarachnoid hemorrhage or bacterial meningitis or bearable headache from chronic increase of intracranial pressure can be examples.

When the meningeal artery is stimulated, the pain location varies depending on the innervating nerves. All 3 divisions of the trigeminal nerve take part in dural innervation.[30] But for intracranial arteries, V1 is the main innervating nerve. In general, pain from stimulating intracranial arteries is referred to the ipsilateral temporal, retrorbital and frontal regions. The pain caused by stimulation of the superior surface of the tentorium, torcular, or straight sinus is also referred to the ipsilateral forehead and periorbital region because this part is innervated by the tentorial nerve from V1.[30]

In a study on balloon inflation of cerebral arteries, balloon inflation produced pain and its location was reproducible. Inflation in the proximal MCA stem produced pain primarily in the ipsilateral temple. Ballooning in the middle of the MCA stem produced pain referred primarily retro-orbitally, and inflation in the distal MCA stem produced pain referred primarily to the forehead.[12] These findings show that there are patterns of pain fiber distribution. Anatomically it is also related to localization of cells of the trigeminal nucleus in the brain stem. Some patients did not perceive any headache with the balloon inflation, which indicates that not all major arteries, or not all parts of major arteries, have pain fibers, and the number of pain receptors may vary by location and among individuals. Stimulation of the superficial temporal and middle meningeal arteries and the large intracranial venous channels can also produce similar referred pain.[10,11,31,32] Therefore, it is natural to think that the precise localization of arterial pain cannot be determined from the location of the pain. One obvious point is a tendency for carotid headaches to be located anteriorly and vertebrobasilar-associated headaches to be located posteriorly.[10,33]

Likewise, pain develops at the posterior neck when the posterior fossa dura is stimulated. It is innervated by the upper 3 cervical spinal nerves. But trigeminal fibers can reach the rostral part of the basilar artery via the posterior communicating artery. The pain from the rostral part of the basilar artery therefore can be referred to the orbital, retro-orbital, and frontal areas. Of interest, sensory signal from the C1 spinal nerve may enter the trigeminal caudal neuclus.[34,35] The nucleus is located from the medulla to the C2 level of the spinal cord, where it continues with the dorsal horn of the spinal cord. The spinal trigeminal tract is also analogous to the Lissauer tract of the spinal cord. One study showed that C1 stimulation produced periorbital and frontal pain.[36] Simultaneous sensitization or interaction between neurons may be the mechanism of common occurrence of both headache and neck pain.[37] Accordingly, pain from the vertebrobasilar system can be perceived as orbital–retro-orbital and frontal pain.[37] Cases of frontal or retro-orbital headaches associated with vertebrobasilar dissection[38] and posterior fossa tumor[39] have been reported. Similarly, sensory fibers from the upper cervical spinal nerve can also reach the distal ICA and neighboring arteries, so pain from the anterior circulation system may also be felt in the posterior neck.[37] In addition, midline crossing fibers that innervate the contralateral side have been noted in both trigeminal and spinal nerves.[40]

Patients with giant aneurysms have plausible reasons for a high incidence of headaches. They have more chance to compress adjacent pain-sensitive structures, including the dura and the artery.[41,42] Traction, compression, and displacement of adjacent arteries produce pain. Pulsatile motion of a large aneurysm sac, thrombus formation within the sac, and extravasation of the thrombin followed by inflammation can also be factors.

Periorbital pain with ptosis from an aneurysm compressing the third nerve is a well-known symptom. Posterior communicating artery aneurysm is the most common cause.[21,43,44] The occulomotor nerve has parasympathetic fibers and motor fibers for eye movement. When a posterior communicating artery aneurysm compresses the third nerve from above, ptosis develops because motor fibers for the levator palpebra muscle are located superficially. The third nerve does not have sensory function, so theoretically pain should not be a symptom unless the pain fibers on the ICA wall is stimulated. However, studies have shown that fibers from V1 of the trigeminal nerve may join and travel with the third nerve at the level of the lateral wall of the cavernous sinus, which accounts for the periorbital pain with third nerve compression.[42]

Some patients with unruptured intracranial aneurysms present with trigeminal neuralgia. Compression or distortion of trigeminal nerves at various levels could be a mechanism. Many aneurysm locations have been reported, including the ICA, posterior cerebral artery, superior cerebellar artery, anterior and posterior inferior cerebellar artery, and basilar artery.[45–47] Typical trigeminal neuralgia involves the V2 and V3 divisions.[48] However, in cases of posterior communicating artery aneurysm associated with trigeminal neuralgia, it mainly occurs in the V1 and V2 area. It is explained by the anatomic location of V1 fibers, which are distributed superiorly and medially in the trigeminal nerve and posterior communicating artery compression of the cavernous sinus from above.[48,49]

The hallmark of subarachnoid hemorrhage (SAH) is a sudden, severe headache. It is often described as head explosion or thunderclap. It is very intense and severe, so many patients describe it as unbearable, or the worst headache of their lives. Typically, it peaks within minutes and last hours or days.[50] In a report, about 50% of the headaches reached a maximum instantaneously. In the others, it took 1 to 5 minutes or longer.[51] In terms of pain location, 70% of the headaches are bilateral. In cases of bilateral headache, generalized headache is most common in 66%. In the case of lateralized headache, frontal and frontoparietal locations are common.[50] Given that a frequent location of ruptured aneurysms is the circle of Willis (anterior circulation) and the subarachnoid space is an open space with bilateral communication, these findings are expected. Meningeal irritation signs, such as nuchal rigidity and the Kernig sign, do not clearly develop at the onset. They take 2 or 3 days to become apparent[52] because development of meningeal inflammation from blood degradation products takes time.

Sentinel headache, which is similar to that of subarachnoid hemorrhage, characterized by sudden severe headache, has been thought to be caused by a small amount of hemorrhage from the aneurysm. When a patient has SAH and the patient has a history of sudden severe headache hours, days, or months before, physicians can consider the previous one to be a sentinel headache. If cerebral aneurysms that will rupture soon could be detected and treated before catastrophic SAH using this warning sign, many patients could be saved.[53] However, real causes of the headaches could be various, including migraine, vasospasm, inflammation, or just tension headache. Other mechanisms, such as acute expansion of the aneurysm, acute formation of a daughter sac, and hemorrhage into the aneurysm wall, can also be considered to be aneurysm-associated sudden severe headache.

Perimesencephalic SAH, a distinct form of SAH with a benign clinical course, is characterized by a small amount of SAH around the midbrain. Angiograms show no source of the bleeding. The cause is thought to be venous or small arterial bleeding.[54] Headache characteristics are not distinct from conventional SAH, which suggests that the real mechanism that produces a sudden severe headache is not necessarily high-pressure bleeding, a large artery rupture hole, or a large subarachnoid hemorrhage. Regardless of pressure, sudden severe headache can develop at the time of rupture of vessels that have pain nerve fibers.

SUMMARY

The pain from an unruptured cerebral aneurysm can occur if it develops in proximal cerebral arteries in which pain fibers are present. These arteries can be the ICA, proximal ACA and MCA, vertebrobasilar arteries, and proximal posterior cerebral artery. Aneurysms at distal arteries do not produce headache unless they stimulate other pain-sensitive structure. The exact level which pain nerve fibers reach on the vessel walls varies between individuals, so some distal aneurysms may produce pain. Slowly formed aneurysms may not induce pain. Rapidly growing or forming aneurysms can cause pain. Acute changes to preexisting aneurysms or arteries can produce pain. Stimulation of larger arterial areas (large aneurysms) possibly causes more pain than small aneurysms.[55] Pain location and characteristics from the aneurysm can be various and nonspecific. The pain-sensing nerves for intracranial structures are the ophthalmic nerve (V1 of the trigeminal nerve) and upper cervical spinal nerves. Maxillary nerves, mandibular nerves, and other minor nerves from VII, IX, and X have sensory function but mainly innervate dura and ear structures. Therefore, pain from supratentorial structures is felt in the orbitofrontal area and that from infratentorial structures is felt at the posterior neck. Pain occurs mostly on the ipsilateral side but some fibers cross-innervate, so bilateral perception may be possible.[21] A sudden severe headache possibly indicates that an acute pain-producing stimulation has occurred. They could include a variety of situations such as rupture of vessels or cerebral aneurysms, tearing (dissection), acute expansion (daughter sac formation), spasm and dilatation (RCVS), embolism (sudden imbedding or stretching of major cerebral arteries by emboli), and migraine. Pain location does not provide decisive information. Diagnosis still depends on the physician's clinical suspicion and work-up.

REFERENCES

1. International Study of Unruptured Intracranial Aneurysms Investigators. Unruptured intracranial aneurysms–risk of rupture and risks of surgical intervention. N Engl J Med 1998;339(24):1725–33.
2. Raps EC, Rogers JD, Galetta SL, et al. The clinical spectrum of unruptured intracranial aneurysms. Arch Neurol 1993;50(3):265–8.
3. Lebedeva ER, Gurary NM, Sakovich VP, et al. Migraine before rupture of intracranial aneurysms. J Headache Pain 2013;14:15.
4. Edvinsson L. Calcitonin gene-related peptide (CGRP) in cerebrovascular disease. ScientificWorldJournal 2002;2:1484–90.
5. Veloso F, Kumar K, Toth C. Headache secondary to deep brain implantation. Headache 1998;38(7):507–15.
6. Goadsby PJ, Lipton RB, Ferrari MD. Migraine–current understanding and treatment. N Engl J Med 2002;346(4):257–70.
7. Tubbs RS, Loukas M, Slappey JB, et al. Clinical anatomy of the C1 dorsal root, ganglion, and ramus: a review and anatomical study. Clin Anat 2007;20(6):624–7.
8. Fontaine D, Almairac F. Pain during awake craniotomy for brain tumor resection. Incidence, causes, consequences and management. Neurochirurgie 2017;63(3):204–7.
9. Wolff DL, Naruse R, Gold M. Nonopioid anesthesia for awake craniotomy: a case report. AANA J 2010;78(1):29–32.
10. Ray B, Wolff H. Experimental studies on headache. Pain sensitive structures of the head and their significance in headache. Arch Surg 1940;41:813–56.
11. Penfield W, McNaughton F. Dural headache and innervation of the dura mater. Arch Neurol Psychiatr 1940;44:43–75.
12. Nichols FT 3rd, Mawad M, Mohr JP, et al. Focal headache during balloon inflation in the internal carotid and middle cerebral arteries. Stroke 1990;21(4):555–9.
13. Nichols FT 3rd, Mawad M, Mohr JP, et al. Focal headache during balloon inflation in the vertebral and basilar arteries. Headache 1993;33(2):87–9.
14. Choi KS, Lee JH, Yi HJ, et al. Incidence and risk factors of postoperative headache after endovascular coil embolization of unruptured intracranial aneurysms. Acta Neurochir (Wien) 2014;156(7):1281–7.
15. Hwang G, Jeong EA, Sohn JH, et al. The characteristics and risk factors of headache development after the coil embolization of an unruptured aneurysm. AJNR Am J Neuroradiol 2012;33(9):1676–8.
16. Fay T. Atypical facial neuralgia, a syndrome of vascular pain. Ann Otol Rhinol Laryngol 1932;41:1030–62.
17. Baron EP, Moskowitz SI, Tepper SJ, et al. Headache following intracranial neuroendovascular procedures. Headache 2012;52(5):739–48.
18. Price DD, McHaffie JG, Larson MA. Spatial summation of heat-induced pain: influence of stimulus area and spatial separation of stimuli on perceived pain sensation intensity and unpleasantness. J Neurophysiol 1989;62(6):1270–9.
19. Staud R, Koo E, Robinson ME, et al. Spatial summation of mechanically evoked muscle pain and painful aftersensations in normal subjects and fibromyalgia patients. Pain 2007;130(1–2):177–87.
20. May A, Buchel C, Turner R, et al. Magnetic resonance angiography in facial and other pain: neurovascular mechanisms of trigeminal sensation. J Cereb Blood Flow Metab 2001;21(10):1171–6.
21. Rodriguez-Catarino M, Frisen L, Wikholm G, et al. Internal carotid artery aneurysms, cranial nerve dysfunction and headache: the role of deformation and pulsation. Neuroradiology 2003;45(4):236–40.
22. Drummond PD, Lance JW. Extracranial vascular changes and the source of pain in migraine headache. Ann Neurol 1983;13(1):32–7.
23. Arndt JO, Klement W. Pain evoked by polymodal stimulation of hand veins in humans. J Physiol 1991;440:467–78.
24. Schwedt TJ, Gereau RW, Frey K, et al. Headache outcomes following treatment of unruptured intracranial aneurysms: a prospective analysis. Cephalalgia 2011;31(10):1082–9.
25. Qureshi AI, Suri MF, Kim SH, et al. Effect of endovascular treatment on headaches in patients with unruptured intracranial aneurysms. Headache 2003;43(10):1090–6.
26. Kong DS, Hong SC, Jung YJ, et al. Improvement of chronic headache after treatment of unruptured

intracranial aneurysms. Headache 2007;47(5): 693–7.

27. Li H, Zhang X, Zhang QR, et al. Resolution of migraine-like headache by coil embolization of a primitive trigeminal artery aneurysm. Pain Med 2014;15(6):1052–5.

28. Choxi AA, Durrani AK, Mericle RA. Both surgical clipping and endovascular embolization of unruptured intracranial aneurysms are associated with long-term improvement in self-reported quantitative headache scores. Neurosurgery 2011;69(1): 128–33 [discussion: 133–4].

29. Gu DQ, Duan CZ, Li XF, et al. Effect of endovascular treatment on headache in elderly patients with unruptured intracranial aneurysms. AJNR Am J Neuroradiol 2013;34(6):1227–31.

30. Wirth FP Jr, Van Buren JM. Referral of pain from dural stimulation in man. J Neurosurg 1971;34(5):630–42.

31. Penfield W. A contribution to the mechanism of intracranial pain. Assoc Res Nerv Ment Dis 1932;15: 399–416.

32. Feindel W, Penfield W, Mc NF. The tentorial nerves and localization of intracranial pain in man. Neurology 1960;10:555–63.

33. Edmeads J. Vascular headaches and the cranial circulation–another look. Headache 1979;19(3): 127–32.

34. Le Doare K, Akerman S, Holland PR, et al. Occipital afferent activation of second order neurons in the trigeminocervical complex in rat. Neurosci Lett 2006; 403(1–2):73–7.

35. Bartsch T, Goadsby PJ. Stimulation of the greater occipital nerve induces increased central excitability of dural afferent input. Brain 2002;125(Pt 7):1496–509.

36. Johnston MM, Jordan SE, Charles AC. Pain referral patterns of the C1 to C3 nerves: implications for headache disorders. Ann Neurol 2013;74(1):145–8.

37. Piovesan EJ, Kowacs PA, Tatsui CE, et al. Referred pain after painful stimulation of the greater occipital nerve in humans: evidence of convergence of cervical afferences on trigeminal nuclei. Cephalalgia 2001;21(2):107–9.

38. Berger MS, Wilson CB. Intracranial dissecting aneurysms of the posterior circulation. Report of six cases and review of the literature. J Neurosurg 1984;61(5):882–94.

39. Kerr RW. A mechanism to account for frontal headache in cases of posterior-fossa tumors. J Neurosurg 1961;18:605–9.

40. Kimmel DL. Innervation of spinal dura mater and dura mater of the posterior cranial fossa. Neurology 1961;11:800–9.

41. Goedee HS, Depauw PR, vd Zwam B, et al. Superficial temporal artery-middle cerebral artery bypass surgery in a pediatric giant intracranial aneurysm presenting as migraine-like episodes. Childs Nerv Syst 2009;25(2):257–61.

42. Hahn CD, Nicolle DA, Lownie SP, et al. Giant cavernous carotid aneurysms: clinical presentation in fifty-seven cases. J Neuroophthalmol 2000;20(4):253–8.

43. Lanzino G, Andreoli A, Tognetti F, et al. Orbital pain and unruptured carotid-posterior communicating artery aneurysms: the role of sensory fibers of the third cranial nerve. Acta Neurochir (Wien) 1993;120(1–2):7–11.

44. Kojo N, Lee S, Otsuru K, et al. A case of ophthalmoplegic migraine with cerebral aneurysm. No Shinkei Geka 1988;16(5 Suppl):503–7 [Japanese].

45. Di Stefano G, Limbucci N, Cruccu G, et al. Trigeminal neuralgia completely relieved after stent-assisted coiling of a superior cerebellar artery aneurysm. World Neurosurg 2017;101:812.e5-9.

46. Ildan F, Gocer AI, Bagdatoglu H, et al. Isolated trigeminal neuralgia secondary to distal anterior inferior cerebellar artery aneurysm. Neurosurg Rev 1996;19(1):43–6.

47. Mendelowitsch A, Radue EW, Gratzl O. Aneurysm, arteriovenous malformation and arteriovenous fistula in posterior fossa compression syndrome. Eur Neurol 1990;30(6):338–42.

48. Sindou M, Leston J, Howeidy T, et al. Micro-vascular decompression for primary trigeminal neuralgia (typical or atypical). Long-term effectiveness on pain; prospective study with survival analysis in a consecutive series of 362 patients. Acta Neurochir (Wien) 2006;148(12):1235–45 [discussion: 1245].

49. Sindou M, Howeidy T, Acevedo G. Anatomical observations during microvascular decompression for idiopathic trigeminal neuralgia (with correlations between topography of pain and site of the neurovascular conflict). Prospective study in a series of 579 patients. Acta Neurochir (Wien) 2002;144(1):1–12 [discussion: 12–3].

50. Al-Shahi R, White PM, Davenport RJ, et al. Subarachnoid haemorrhage: lumbar puncture for every negative scan? Authors' reply. BMJ 2006;333(7567):550.

51. Linn FH, Rinkel GJ, Algra A, et al. Headache characteristics in subarachnoid haemorrhage and benign thunderclap headache. J Neurol Neurosurg Psychiatry 1998;65(5):791–3.

52. Sarner M, Rose F. Clinical presentation of ruptured intracranial aneurysm. J Neurol Neurosurg Psychiatry 1967;30:67–70.

53. Polmear A. Sentinel headaches in aneurysmal subarachnoid haemorrhage: what is the true incidence? A systematic review. Cephalalgia 2003;23(10): 935–41.

54. van Gijn J, van Dongen KJ, Vermeulen M, et al. Perimesencephalic hemorrhage: a nonaneurysmal and benign form of subarachnoid hemorrhage. Neurology 1985;35(4):493–7.

55. Ji W, Liu A, Yang X, et al. Incidence and predictors of headache relief after endovascular treatment in patients with unruptured intracranial aneurysms. Interv Neuroradiol 2017;23(1):18–27.

The Connection Between Patent Foramen Ovale and Migraine

Preetham Kumar, MD[a], Yasufumi Kijima, MD, PhD[b],
Brian H. West, MD, MS[a], Jonathan M. Tobis, MD[a],*

KEYWORDS

• Migraine headache • Patent foramen ovale • Right-to-left shunt

KEY POINTS

• Although observational studies have shown that migraineurs with aura respond well to patent foramen ovale (PFO) closure, randomized trials have not confirmed this.
• Until a randomized double-blinded study clearly demonstrates a significant benefit of PFO closure to reduce migraines, medical therapy will remain the treatment of choice for migraines.
• One challenge in conducting such a study is adequate patient recruitment in a timely fashion given strict inclusion criteria.

BACKGROUND

A patent foramen ovale (PFO) is a remnant of the fetal circulation that permits oxygenated blood from the placenta to pass from the inferior vena cava across the atrial septum into the arterial circulation (Fig. 1). This mechanism of bypassing the nonfunctional fetal lungs and directing oxygenated blood to the fetal brain is critical for fetal development and is preserved by evolution in all mammals. After birth, the lungs are aerated and serve to oxygenate the blood; the pressure in the left atrium exceeds that in the right atrium and the septum primum closes over the foramen ovale and fuses with the septum secundum. By genetically determined mechanisms,[1] the foramen ovale remains patent in 20% to 30% of the general adult population. Thus, PFO is by far the most common congenital heart defect. Although most people with a PFO remain asymptomatic, in people who have migraine with aura, the presence of a PFO is about 50%.[2] One hypothesis for this 2-fold higher frequency of PFO is that a genetic influence might predispose some patients to a higher risk of developing both

migraine and atrial septal abnormalities. Another hypothesis is that migraine, especially migraine with aura, may be triggered by vasoactive substances (eg, serotonin) that are ordinarily metabolized during passage through the lungs, and the presence of a right-to-left shunt such as a PFO or a pulmonary arteriovenous malformation allows these chemicals to bypass metabolic alteration in the lungs and gain entry to the arterial circulation in a higher concentration so that on reaching the brain, they stimulate receptors in susceptible individuals, which produces the cerebral migraine phenomena. The latter hypothesis was derived after the observation that PFO closure often resulted in relief of migraine headaches (Figs. 2–5).

OBSERVATIONAL STUDIES SUGGESTING AN ASSOCIATION BETWEEN MIGRAINE AND PATENT FORAMEN OVALE

In 1998, Del Sette and colleagues at the University of Genova, Italy, described the first association between right-to-left shunting, stroke, and migraine with aura. Del Sette and colleagues

[a] Cardiology, University of California, Los Angeles, Room B-976 Factor Building, Box # 951717, Los Angeles, CA 90095-1717, USA; [b] Department of Cardiovascular Medicine, St. Luke's International Hospital, 9-1 Akaishi-cho, Chuo-ku, Tokyo 104-8560, Japan
* Corresponding author.
E-mail address: Jtobis@mednet.ucla.edu

Neuroimag Clin N Am 29 (2019) 261–270
https://doi.org/10.1016/j.nic.2019.01.006

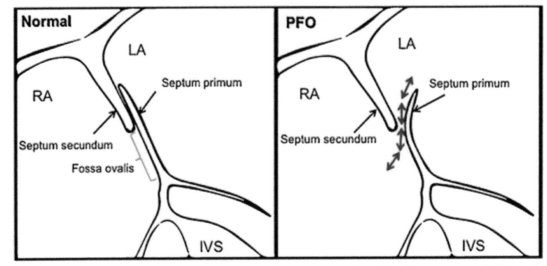

Fig. 1. PFO anatomy. IVS, interventricular septum; LA, left atrium; RA, right atrium. (*From* Yasunaga D, Hamon M. MDCT of interatrial septum. Diagn Interv Imaging 2015;96:893; with permission.)

carried out a case-control study in which 44 patients suffering from migraine with aura, 73 patients younger than 50 year with a history of cryptogenic focal cerebral ischemia, and 50 controls asymptomatic for cerebrovascular disease and without a history of migraine underwent bilateral transcranial Doppler (TCD) with injection of contrast medium during normal ventilation and during Valsalva maneuver. The prevalence of a right to left shunt was 41% (18/44) in patients with migraine with aura and 35% (26/73) in patients with cryptogenic stroke, compared with 16% (8/50) in normal controls (P<.005).[3]

Schwedt and colleagues[4] conducted a systematic review of case-control studies published up to 2008 looking at PFO and migraines and concluded that there is a bidirectional association. Migraine

with aura (but not without aura) is more common in patients with PFO than in the general population, and PFO is more prevalent in patients who have migraine with aura than in the general population. Anzola and colleagues[5] compared the frequency of right-to-left shunt using TCD in 113 patients who had migraine with aura, 53 patients who had migraine without aura, and 25 age-matched controls. PFO was present in 48% of subjects who had migraine with aura, but was not different in migraineurs without aura (23%), compared with the control group without migraine (20%) (P = .002).

Wilmshurst and colleagues[6] were the first to report the benefits of PFO closure on migraine headache. Of 37 patients who underwent PFO closure, 21 (57%) had a history of migraines, with 16 having a history of migraine with aura and 5

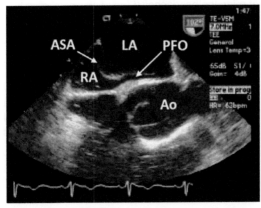

Fig. 2. Transesophageal echocardiography showing a long-tunnel PFO with an atrial septal aneurysm (ASA). Ao, aorta; LA, left atrium; RA, right atrium.

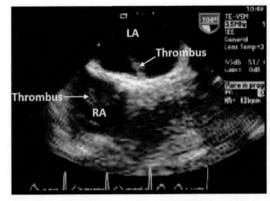

Fig. 3. A thrombus caught straddling the PFO between the right and left atrium. LA, left atrium; RA, right atrium.

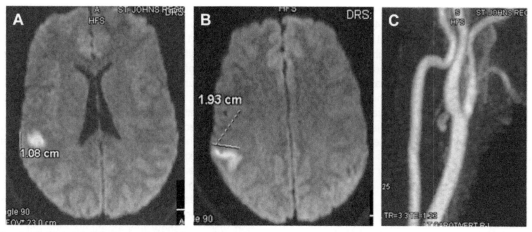

Fig. 4. (*A, B*) Axial diffusion-weighted images showing a 1.08 × 1.93 cm cortical infarct. (*C*) MR angiogram of the neck showing patent carotid arteries.

having a history of migraine without aura. Following PFO closure, 7 out of 16 (44%) migraineurs with aura had complete resolution of migraines and 8 of the remaining 9 had an improvement in both frequency and severity of migraines, whereas 3 out of 5 (60%) migraineurs without aura had complete resolution of migraines.

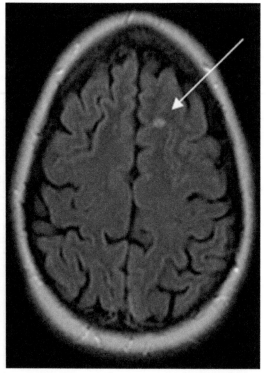

Fig. 5. Brain MR imaging of a patient with frequent migraines who had white matter lesions. *Arrow* identifies white matter lesion visible on FLAIR axial image.

Khessali and colleagues[7] assessed the prevalence of right-to-left shunt in patients with visual aura and evaluated the effect of shunt closure on resolution of aura. The investigators divided the study population into 2 groups, one group with visual aura (n = 225) and the other group as the control (n = 200). The visual aura group was further subdivided into 3 subgroups. Group A (n = 175) consisted of patients who had a history of visual aura that was followed by a migraine headache immediately or within 60 mins. Group B (n = 29) consisted of patients with a history of visual aura and migraine headache that were temporally unrelated (ie, not occurring within 60 mins of each other). Group C (n = 21) consisted of patients with a history of visual aura without a history of headache. In the 3 groups, 168 (96%, *P*<.0001), 21 (72%, *P*<.0001), and 14 (67%, *P*<.0001) patients were positive for right-to-left shunt, respectively. PFO closure was performed in 67 (40%), 8 (38%), and 5 (36%) patients within each group, respectively; and 52% (35/67), 75% (6/8), and 80% (4/5) had complete resolution of visual aura at the 12-month follow-up. The similar distribution of right-to-left shunt in all 3 patient groups and the correlation between PFO closure and improvement of aura suggests a similar pathophysiology between the presence of PFO and the visual aura phenomenon, regardless of whether headache is present in the symptom complex.

In contrast to the findings of the above mentioned studies, Rundek and colleagues[8] conducted a population-based study in which 1101 patients with a history of migraines were evaluated for PFO using transthoracic echocardiography (TTE) with saline contrast and provocative maneuvers and the investigators did not find a significant difference in the prevalence of PFO among subjects who had migraine compared with those who did not have migraine (14.6% vs 15%). It is important to understand that the frequency of finding a right-to-left shunt highly depends on the type of testing that is performed. TTE has a 40% false-negative rate, TEE has a 10% false-negative rate, and TCD is the most sensitive noninvasive test with a 3% false-negative rate when all 3 studies are compared with a diagnostic right heart catheterization and probing the atrial septum with a guidewire.[9]

The aforementioned studies are summarized in Table 1.

RANDOMIZED CLINICAL TRIALS SUGGESTING AN ASSOCIATION BETWEEN MIGRAINE AND PATENT FORAMEN OVALE

The previous studies were all observational and subject to recognized bias of nonrandomized data. The MIST (Migraine Intervention with STAR-Flex Technology) trial was the first to investigate the effects of PFO closure for migraine in a prospective, randomized, double-blind, sham-controlled clinical trial. Patients who suffered from migraine with aura, experienced frequent migraine attacks, had more than or equal to 2 previously failed classes of prophylactic treatments, and had a moderate or large right-to-left shunt consistent with the presence of a PFO were randomized to transcatheter PFO closure with the STARFlex implant or to a sham procedure. One hundred forty-seven patients were randomized

and followed for 6 months. The primary efficacy end point was complete cessation of migraine headache 91 to 180 days after the procedure. No significant difference was observed in the primary end point of migraine headache cessation between implant and sham groups (3/74 vs 3/73, respectively; $P = .51$). The secondary efficacy end point was the frequency of migraine headache days. The reduction in migraine days was not statistically significant. Two hypotheses were developed to explain why the MIST trial did not achieve the expected success and dramatic reduction in frequency of migraine headaches that was described in the observational studies. The first hypothesis stated that the patient population was somehow fundamentally different on a mechanistic or physiologic basis than the patient populations that were treated in the observational studies. The second hypothesis stated that the right to left shunt in the study population was not effectively closed by the particular device used.[10]

The PREMIUM (Prospective, Randomized Investigation to Evaluate Incidence of Headache Reduction in Subjects with Migraine and PFO Using the AMPLATZER PFO Occluder to Medical Management) trial was a double-blind study investigating migraine characteristics for more than 1 year in subjects randomized to medical therapy and PFO closure with the Amplatzer PFO Occluder device (Abbott Vascular, Chicago) versus medical therapy and a sham procedure (right heart catheterization). Subjects had to have 6 to 14 days of migraine per month, had failed at least 3 migraine

Table 1
Observational studies of the prevalence of migraine in patients referred for PFO closure and the effect of the procedure on migraine

Study	Prevalence of Migraine in Patients Referred for PFO Closure	% Migraine Improved/ Cured Following PFO Closure	Length of Follow-up (mo)
Wilmshurst et al,[32] 2000	21/37 (57%)	86	30
Morandi et al,[33] 2003	17/62 (27%)	88	6
Schwerzmann et al,[34] 2004	48/215 (22%)	81	12
Post et al,[35] 2004	26/66 (39%)	65	6
Reisman et al,[36] 2005	57/162 (35%)	70	12
Azarbal et al,[37] 2005	37/89 (42%)	76	18
Donti et al,[38] 2006	35/131 (27%)	91	20
Anzola et al,[39] 2006	50/163 (31%)	88	12
Kimmelstiel et al,[40] 2007	24/41 (59%)	83	3
Papa et al,[41] 2009	28/76 (37%)	82	12
Khessali et al,[7] 2012	204/590 (35%)	76	12
Total	547/1632 (34%)	80.5	13 ± 7.5

preventive medications, and had a significant right-to-left shunt defined by TCD grade 4 or 5. Of 1653 subjects consented, 230 were enrolled. The primary efficacy endpoint was responder rate (defined as 50% reduction in migraine attacks). The primary endpoint was achieved in 45/117 (38.5%) patients randomized to device and 33/103 (32%) patients randomized to control, failing to show statistical significance ($P = .32$). The secondary efficacy endpoint was reduction in migraine days. The study group experienced migraines less often than the control group and the difference was statistically significant (-3.4 vs -2.0 d/mo, $P = .025$). In addition, 10 of 117 patients (8.5%) who underwent PFO closure had complete migraine remission by 1 year versus 1 (1%) in the control group ($P = .01$). Although the PREMIUM trial did not demonstrate efficacy for PFO closure using the primary endpoint of responder rate, an additional subset analysis was performed that evaluated subjects who had aura as a consistent component of their migraine attacks (aura present in >50% of migraine episodes). For this subgroup analysis, there was a significant difference in the responder rate: 49% (19 of 39) versus 23% (9 of 40) for device versus control group, respectively ($P = .015$). In addition, for subjects with frequent aura, 15.4% (6 of 39) had complete cessation of their migraine attacks versus 2.5% (1 of 40) in the control group ($P = .04$). The potential benefit in a minority of migraine patients suggests a need to further investigate populations who are more likely to benefit from PFO closure than the medication refractory population.[11] It is expected that future trials will focus on PFO closure in a more select patient population of migraine with frequent aura.

The PRIMA (Percutaneous closure of patent foramen ovale in migraine with aura) trial was a multicenter, prospective, randomized, open-label international trial that evaluated if percutaneous PFO closure was effective in reducing migraine headaches in patients with migraine with aura that were refractory to medical treatment. Participants had to be diagnosed with migraine before the age of 50, had to experience more than or equal to 3 migraine attacks or more than or equal to 5 migraine headache days per month and less than 15 migraine days per month over the 3 months preceding enrollment, and had to be unresponsive to 2 commonly prescribed preventive medications. Of 705 subjects screened over a 90-day screening period involving 3 screening visits, 107 were enrolled. The enrolled patients were subsequently randomized 1:1 to either percutaneous PFO closure (n = 53) or medical management (n = 54) and then followed for 12 months. Of

note, within 14 days of randomization, both groups were given acetylsalicylic acid 75 to 100 mg/d for 6 months and clopidogrel 75 mg/d for 3 months. The primary efficacy endpoint was reduction in monthly migraine days during months 9 to 12 after randomization compared with months 1 to 3 before randomization. Although the PFO closure group experienced less migraine days per month than the control group, the difference was not significant (-2.9 vs -1.7 days, respectively, $P = .17$). The secondary efficacy endpoint was average reduction in migraine attacks and although the PFO closure group experienced less migraine attacks than the control group, the difference was not significant (-2.1 attacks vs -1.3 attacks, respectively, $P = .097$). Four of forty patients (10%) in the PFO closure group were completely free of migraine attacks during months 10 to 12 compared with 0 of 41 patients (0%) in the control group but this was not significant ($P = .055$). Neither antiplatelet agent had significant influence on headache days. Although the PRIMA trial failed to show that PFO closure significantly reduced overall monthly migraine days compared with ongoing medical management in patients with refractory migraine with aura and PFO, a post hoc analysis focusing solely on migraines with aura showed that the number of migraine with aura days and migraine with aura attacks were markedly reduced in the PFO closure group compared with controls (-2.4 vs -0.6 days, respectively, [$P = .0141$] and -2.0 vs -0.5 attacks, respectively, [$P = .0003$]). In addition, 16 of 40 patients (40%) in the PFO closure group were completely free of migraine attacks with aura compared with 4 of 40 patients (10%) in the control group ($P = .004$). These latter findings support the hypothesis that PFOs play a major role in pathogenicity for migraine with aura. In stroke, the ROPE score is used to determine if a PFO is stroke related or incidental. Similarly, it is theorized that the presence or absence of aura can resolve the question of incidental versus pathogenic PFO. Limitations to the trial include lack of blinding of the PRIMA patients, premature termination of the study by the sponsor due to slow enrollment, due to slow enrollment, lack of a sham intervention, and failure to completely abolish the right-to-left shunts in 12% of the PFO closure group.[12]

ASSOCIATION OF PATENT FORAMEN OVALE, MIGRAINE, AND CRYPTOGENIC STROKE

People who have migraine headache, especially migraineurs with aura, have an increased risk of cryptogenic stroke.[13] Cryptogenic stroke, or stroke of unknown cause, is a diagnosis of exclusion after standard causes of stroke have been ruled out by an extensive workup. This definition typically applies to people younger than 60 years, above which it is assumed that atherosclerosis is present and is the most likely cause of the stroke. The origin of the thrombus is usually not found unless a peripheral deep vein thrombosis is present. It is hypothesized that one cause of cryptogenic stroke is a venous thrombus, perhaps from peripheral or pelvic varicose veins, that bypasses the lungs via a PFO and enters the arterial circulation. Occasionally, this paradoxic embolism can be documented by echocardiography when a large thrombus trapped in a PFO (Fig. 3). The venous clots that produce cryptogenic stroke are usually less than 3 mm in diameter. However, once the clot passes to the brain, it is not possible to prove how it got there.

According to a meta-analysis of 6 case-control studies, the relative risk (RR) of ischemic stroke for migraine with aura and migraine without aura are 2.3 and 1.8, respectively. The RR of ischemic stroke in women with migraine using oral contraceptives is increased to 8.7, suggesting that women with migraine should not take oral contraceptives.[14] One study in the Netherlands used MR imaging to assess 134 patients who had migraine without aura, 61 patients who had migraine with aura, and 140 matched controls. Although the total percentage of patients with an ischemic infarct was not increased in migraineurs versus controls (5% vs 8.1%), when the data were analyzed by vascular supply, there was an increased incidence of posterior circulation infarcts in migraineurs with aura (8.1% vs 0.7%).[15]

In Iceland, the Age Gene/Environment Susceptibility (AGES) – Reykjavík study prospectively observed 4689 people for an average of 25 years and then performed a brain MR imaging. Migraine was present in 12.2% of the participants and 63% of this subgroup was identified as having migraine with aura. Patients who had migraine with aura had an increased risk of subsequent infarct lesions on MR imaging (OR 1.4; 95% CI 1.1–1.8). However, because the study did not assess for the presence of right-to-left shunting, we do not know the relative frequency of PFO in those migraineurs who developed stroke versus the migraineurs who did not develop a stroke.[16]

According to the initial theory of migraines and aura, it was believed that migraine was "a vascular headache" due to ischemia caused by intense arterial vasospasm. It was also thought that if the arterial constriction was prolonged and severe enough, a cerebral infarct could ensue. Over time, the understanding of the cause of migraine has changed. Several lines of evidence, including functional MR imaging, PET imaging during migraine, and gene insertion studies of familial migraine with hemiplegia in mice, demonstrate that migraine is initiated by vasodilation and then vasoconstriction (not the converse), but the severity of decreased flow is about 25%, which is not sufficient to induce an infarct. The current theory is that migraine represents neurovascular dysfunction associated with allodynia (painful response to any stimuli) involving multiple areas within the brain. The transient neurologic deficits, manifested as aura, are due to a spreading wave of depolarization over the cerebral cortex (cortical spreading depression [CSD]) that starts in the occipital area and progresses over the sensory and motor cortex at 2 to 3 mm/min. The aura sequence corresponds to the timing of the CSD and usually lasts 20 minutes. The question remains, why is there a higher prevalence of stroke in migraineurs? One possibility is that there is an association of migraine with accelerated atherosclerosis, but there has never been any evidence to demonstrate this metabolic hypothesis.

The prevalence of migraine headache in people who present with cryptogenic stroke is approximately 30% to 50%. Both migraine with aura and cryptogenic stroke are associated with a higher frequency of PFO. So, in people with migraine headaches who develop stroke, what is the frequency of right-to-left shunting? Wilmshurst and colleagues[17] demonstrated that the prevalence of a right-to-left shunt in patients with a history of migraine with aura who had a stroke (84%) was significantly greater compared with patients with a history of migraine with aura but no history of stroke (38.1%, P<.001), patients without a history of migraine who had a stroke (55.6%, P<.05), and population controls (12.2%, P<.001). In addition, the prevalence of right-to-left shunt in patients with a history of migraine without aura who had a stroke (75%) was also significantly greater compared with patients who had migraine with aura but no history of stroke (38.1%, P<.05) and population controls (12.2%, P<.001). This observation led to the theory that the increased frequency of stroke in migraineurs is due to the presence of a PFO for both conditions: the PFO is the pathway through which the migraine with aura is chemically triggered and also increases the likelihood of having a paradoxic embolism pass from the venous side to the brain.

This theory is also consistent with the higher risk of stroke in migraineurs who are on birth control pills or hormone replacement therapy.[18] Estrogen increases the risk of venous thrombosis. If a PFO is present, as suggested by the history of migraine with aura, it is possible that a venous thrombus, induced by the addition of estrogen, may permit a paradoxic embolism to occur and result in a cryptogenic stroke. If this hypothesis can be confirmed, the next step would be evaluation of prophylactic closure of PFO in a randomized trial to test whether it is an effective method of treatment for prevention of stroke in migraineurs. However, this type of study would be difficult to perform as the absolute risk of stroke in migraineurs is small. Therefore, a large number of patients would need to be treated with PFO closure and followed-up over many years to show an effect.

Between January 2008 and November 2017, the UCLA Comprehensive Stroke Center identified 712 patients with ischemic stroke; 127 patients (18%) were diagnosed as having a cryptogenic stroke. Of these, 68 patients had adequate testing for PFO and a documented migraine history. Of the 34 patients with both cryptogenic stroke and migraines, 27 (79%) had a PFO. Of the 15 patients with cryptogenic stroke and migraine with frequent aura, 14 (93%) had a PFO. Of the 34 patients with cryptogenic stroke but without a history of migraines, 20 (59%) had a PFO. The difference in prevalence of PFO between patients with cryptogenic stroke with migraine, with migraine with aura, and without migraine was statistically significant ($P = .042$). When compared with a control general population of 200 people where the prevalence of PFO was 18%, patients with cryptogenic stroke with or without migraine had significantly greater prevalence of PFO ($P<.00001$ and $P<.00001$, respectively).[13] These observations suggest that the majority (60%) of cryptogenic strokes are associated with a PFO and that the strokes that occur in migraineurs with aura are almost always associated with a PFO.

ASSOCIATION OF MIGRAINE AND FLOW RATE ACROSS A PATENT FORAMEN OVALE

A retrospective study in 142 migraine subjects looked at the relationship between the degree of right-to-left shunt and visual aura. Eighty-two (58%) subjects were classified into the frequent aura (aura present in >50% of migraine attacks) group, and 60 (42%) were classified into the occasional (≤50%) or no aura group. The degree of right-to-left shunt was measured by TCD using the Spencer Logarithmic Scale, which assigns a score of 0 to 5, with grade 3 or higher considered as a positive result representing a significant right-to-left shunt. TCD Spencer grade in the frequent aura group was significantly greater than that in the occasional or no aura group both at rest and post-Valsalva (3.2 ± 1.4 vs 2.1 ± 1.6, $P<.001$ for

rest; 4.3 ± 1.0 vs 3.8 ± 1.3, $P = .009$ for post-Valsalva). Therefore, migraineurs who have frequent visual aura have a greater degree of right-to-left shunt than migraineurs with infrequent visual aura.[19] This observation that the degree of right-to-left shunting affects the frequency of migraine aura demonstrates that there is a dose-response effect between PFO flow and aura frequency.

MIGRAINE AND CEREBRAL WHITE MATTER LESIONS

Migraineurs have a higher frequency of white matter lesions (WML) in the brain detected by MR imaging.[20] WML are usually 2 to 5 mm hyperintense signals appearing on FLAIR or T2 sequences that are secondary to axonal degeneration, gliosis, and demyelination believed to be the result of microvascular ischemia (see Fig. 5). WML can be detected anywhere along the white matter tracts of the cerebrum, cerebellum, and the brainstem. WML appear similar to lesions found in multiple sclerosis, vasculitis, and lacunar strokes. It is not clear why migraineurs should have a higher incidence of WML, but the assumption has been that migraine produces vascular constriction and ischemia that could damage the axonal myelin. A second possibility is that migraine stimulates a metabolic process that is detrimental to the myelin sheath.

In one study from France, 1643 individuals older than 65 years had WML on MR imaging and were followed-up for 5 years. The risk of developing a subsequent stroke in these patients was directly correlated with the volume of the WML and was 5 times higher for the highest quartile of WML volume. However, the presence of WML did not predict other cardiovascular outcomes, suggesting that the pathophysiology of WML may be different from large vessel atherosclerosis.[21] The presence of a PFO was not assessed in this population.

Another theory for the presence of WML in migraineurs is ischemic insult associated with a right-to-left shunt due to embolic material such as platelet clumps that could bypass filtration in the lungs and enter the cerebral circulation. An Italian group headed by Carlo Vigna conducted an observational study of 82 patients, all of whom had a PFO, severe migraine, and WML on MR imaging. All 82 patients were offered PFO closure and 53 patients elected to undergo a PFO closure procedure. In the subjects who had their PFO closed, the number of migraine attacks was reduced from 32 ± 9 in the 6 months before closure to 7 ± 7 in the 6 months after closure ($P<.001$). In the 29 subjects who elected not to undergo PFO closure, there was no significant reduction in migraines (from 36 ± 13 to 30 ± 21). This study suggests that migraineurs with WML may identify a group that is particularly sensitive to PFO closure. It also suggests that in some people, the presence of a PFO could be causally related to WML. However, it is unclear whether this is because PFO is casually related to migraine, or whether the WML are a sign of greater responsiveness to PFO closure.[22] In addition, this was an observational study and not a randomized trial.

Data supporting this hypothesis have been conflicting. Bosca and colleagues[23] imaged 44 migraineurs with and without aura; 29 patients (66%) had WML but only 7 of the 29 (24%) patients with WML had a right-to-left shunt. This suggests either that there are multiple causes for WML in migraine or that right-to-left shunting is unrelated to WML. Del Sette and colleagues[24] conducted a similar study with 80 patients and arrived at the same conclusion.

In support of the theory that migraine produces WML is the observation that migraineurs without a PFO have a high incidence of WML on MR imaging.[23,24] But WML also are present in people with PFO who do not have migraine. This is a difficult area to study, because there is an increase in WML with increasing age, so that comparison studies need to adjust for the age of the subjects. In addition, it is difficult to obtain a control population of people who are asymptomatic but have had a brain MR imaging. There are several open-access repositories of brain MR imaging in a normal population.[25] The prevalence of WML per decade was looked at in subjects with a known right-to-left shunt versus this control general population (Yasufumi Kijima, MD and Jonathan M. Tobis, MD, unpublished data, 2016). There were 397 subjects who had a documented right-to-left shunt using TCD with bubble contrast who underwent brain MR imaging. These subjects were then divided into migraineur (N = 244) and non-migraineur (N = 153) groups. Between 20 and 60 years of age, in nonmigraineurs with a right-to-left shunt, WML were more prevalent compared with age-matched controls. However, in people aged 60 to 80 years, the incidence of WML in non-migraineurs with known right-to-left shunt was no greater than that of the general elderly population. Within each 2 decade age group of migraineurs with a right-to-left shunt (group A), nonmigraineurs with a right-to-left shunt (group B), and the control subjects (group C), WML were more prevalent in migraineurs versus controls in 2 age groups: 20 to 39 years (27% vs 13% vs 10%, P<.01) and 40 to 59 years (58% vs 47% vs 30%, P<.001). However, WML were also more prevalent than controls

in the group with a right-to-left shunt but without migraine in the 40 to 59 year olds. This observation suggests that both migraine without a right-to-left shunt and a right-to-left shunt without migraine may predispose to the development of WML. The results of prior studies may vary if they did not take into account the age of the subjects.

One concern regarding the presence of WML is the long-term consequences. To date, WML have been linked to strokes, cognitive impairment, and dementia but some of these links have conflicting evidence. In regard to stroke, a 2010 meta-analysis of 12 studies looking at the association of white matter hyperintensities with risk of first ever stroke demonstrated a significant association between the 2 (hazard ratio [HR] 3.3, 95% CI: 2.6–4.4, P<.001).[26] Furthermore, a pooled population-based analysis of the Atherosclerosis Risk in Communities Study and Cardiovascular Health Study (CHS), which followed 4872 clinically stroke-free individuals over a median of 13 years, demonstrated that greater MR imaging–defined burden of WML was a risk factor for spontaneous intraparenchymal hemorrhage (P<.0001).[27] In regard to cognitive impairment, a study looking at 67 American participants with normal cognition found that high baseline WML was related to the risk of progression to mild cognitive impairment (MCI) (HR 3.3; 95% CI 1.33–8.2, P = .01) but the Framingham Offspring Study, which observed 1694 participants for a mean duration of 6.2 years, showed that the volume of WML was associated with risk of MCI only in those aged 60 years or older (OR 1.49, 95% CI: 1.14–1.97, P<.05).[28,29] Lastly, other studies, showed that the burden of WML was significantly associated with an increased risk of dementia.[29,30]

THE PATHWAY FORWARD

Although observational studies have shown that migraineurs with aura respond well to PFO closure, randomized trials have not confirmed this. Until a randomized double-blinded study clearly demonstrates a significant benefit of PFO closure to reduce migraines, medical therapy will remain the treatment of choice for migraines. One challenge in conducting such a study is adequate patient recruitment in a timely fashion given strict inclusion criteria. For example, a large number of patients who were screened for MIST II were excluded because the number of headache days exceeded the upper cutoff for the trial. Another challenge is finding patients with similar clinical characteristics to those who benefitted from PFO closure in the observational studies. Often, these patients presented with migraine and frequent aura or cryptogenic stroke. Another proposal has been to enroll patients who respond to antiplatelet therapy.[31] The authors are optimistic that a future randomized trial of PFO closure to reduce migraine will identify the correct patient subset, and PFO closure will become part of the treatment options for people who suffer from migraine.

REFERENCES

1. Wilmshurst P, Nightingale S. Relationship between migraine and cardiac and pulmonary right-to-left shunts. Clin Sci 2001;100:215–20.

2. Niessen K, Karsan A. Notch signaling in the developing cardiovascular system. Am J Physiol Cell Physiol 2007;293(1):C1–11.

3. Del Sette M, Angeli S, Leandri M, et al. Migraine with aura and right-to-left shunt on transcranial Doppler: a case-control study. Cerebrovasc Dis 1998;8:327.

4. Schwedt TJ, Demaerschalk BM, Dodick DW. Patent foramen ovale and migraine: a quantitative systematic review. Cephalalgia 2008;28:531.

5. Anzola GP, Magoni M, Guindani M, et al. Potential source of cerebral embolism in migraine with aura: a trans-cranial Doppler study. Neurology 1999;52(8):1622–5.

6. Wilmshurst PT, Pearson MJ, Nightingale S, et al. Inheritance of persistent foramen ovale and atrial septal defects and the relation to familial migraine with aura. Heart 2004;90(11):1315–20.

7. Khessali H, Mojadidi MK, Gevorgyan R, et al. The effect of patent foramen ovale closure on visual aura without headache or typical aura with migraine headache. JACC Cardiovasc Interv 2012;5(6):682–7.

8. Rundek T, Elkind MS, Di Tullio MR, et al. Patent foramen ovale and migraine: a cross-sectional study from the Northern Manhattan Study (NOMAS). Circulation 2008;118:1419.

9. Mojadidi MK, Roberts SC, Winoker JS, et al. Accuracy of transcranial Doppler for the diagnosis of intracardiac right-to-left shunt: a bivariate meta-analysis of prospective studies. JACC Cardiovasc Imaging 2014;7(3):236–50.

10. Dowson A, Mullen M, Peatfield R, et al. Migraine intervention with STARFlex technology (MIST) trial. Circulation 2008;117(11):1397–404.

11. Tobis J, Charles A, Silberstein SD, et al. Percutaneous closure of patent foramen ovale in patients with migraine: the PREMIUM trial. J Am Coll Cardiol 2017;70(22):2766–74.

12. Mattle HP, Evers S, Hildick-Smith D, et al. Percutaneous closure of patent foramen ovale in migraine with aura, a randomized controlled trial. Eur Heart J 2016;37:2029–36.

13. West BH, Noureddin N, Mamzhi Y, et al. Frequency of patent foramen ovale and migraine in patients with cryptogenic stroke. Stroke 2018;49(5):1123–8.

14. Etminan M, Takkouche B, Isorna FC, et al. Risk of ischaemic stroke in people with migraine: systematic review and meta-analysis of observational studies. BMJ 2005;330(7482):63.

15. Kruit MC, van Buchem MA, Hofman PA, et al. Migraine as a risk factor for subclinical brain lesions. JAMA 2004;291(4):427–34.

16. Scher AI, Gudmundsson LS, Sigurdsson S, et al. Migraine headache in middle age and late-life brain infarcts. JAMA 2009;301(24):2564–70.

17. Wilmshurst P, Nightingale S, Pearson M, et al. Relation of atrial shunts to migraine in patients with ischemic stroke and peripheral emboli. Am J Cardiol 2006;98(6):831–3.

18. MacGregor EA. Estrogen replacement and migraine. Maturitas 2009;63(1):51–5.

19. Kijima Y, Miller N, Noureddin N, et al. The degree of right-to-left shunt is associated with visual aura due to migraine. J Am Coll Cardiol 2015;66(15):TCT–738.

20. Kruit M, Buchem MV, Launer L, et al. Migraine is associated with an increased risk of deep white matter lesions, subclinical posterior circulation infarcts and brain iron accumulation: the population-based MRI CAMERA study. Cephalalgia 2010;30(2):129–36.

21. Buyck JF, Dufouil C, Mazoyer B, et al. Cerebral white matter lesions are associated with the risk of stroke but not with other vascular events: the 3-City Dijon Study. Stroke 2009;40(7):2327–31.

22. Vigna C, Marchese N, Inchingolo V, et al. Improvement of migraine after patent foramen ovale percutaneous closure in patients with subclinical brain lesions: a case-control study. JACC Cardiovasc Interv 2009;2(2):107–13.

23. Bosca M, Tembl J, Bosca I, et al. Study of the relationship between white matter lesions in the magnetic resonance imaging and patent foramen ovale. Neurologia 2008;23(8):499–502.

24. Sette MD, Dinia L, Bonzano L, et al. White matter lesions in migraine and right-to-left shunt: a conventional and diffusion MRI study. Cephalalgia 2008;28(4):376–82.

25. Job DE, Dickie DA, Rodriquez D, et al. A brain imaging repository of normal structural MRI across the life course: brain images of normal subjects (BRAINS). Neuroimage 2017;144(B):200–304.

26. Debette S, Markus HS. The clinical importance of white matter hyperintensities on brain magnetic resonance imaging: systematic review and meta-analysis. BMJ 2010;341:c3666.

27. Folsom AR, Yatsuya H, Mosley TH Jr, et al. Risk of intraparenchymal hemorrhage with magnetic

resonance imaging-defined leukoaraiosis and brain infarcts. Ann Neurol 2012;71:552–9.

28. Smith EE, Egorova S, Blacker D, et al. Magnetic resonance imaging white matter hyperintensities and brain volume in the prediction of mild cognitive impairment and dementia. Arch Neurol 2008;65: 94–100.

29. Debette S, Beiser A, DeCarli C, et al. Association of MRI markers of vascular brain injury with incident stroke, mild cognitive impairment, dementia, and mortality: the Framingham Offspring Study. Stroke 2010;41:600–6.

30. Kuller LH, Lopez OL, Newman A, et al. Risk factors for dementia in the cardiovascular health cognition study. Neuroepidemiology 2003;22:13–22.

31. Sommer RJ. PFO closure for migraine: dead, alive, or in need of another trial? Denver (CO): TCT; 2017.

32. Wilmshurst PT, Nightingale S, Walsh KP, et al. Effect on migraine of closure of cardiac right-to-left shunts to prevent recurrence of decompression illness or stroke or for haemodynamic reasons. Lancet 2000; 356(9242):1648–51.

33. Morandi E, Anzola GP, Angeli S, et al. Transcatheter closure of patent foramen ovale: a new migraine treatment? J Interv Cardiol 2003;16(1):39–42.

34. Schwerzmann M, Wiher S, Nedeltchev K, et al. Percutaneous closure of patent foramen ovale reduces the frequency of migraine attacks. Neurology 2004;62(8):1399–401.

35. Post MC, Thijs V, Herroelen L, et al. Closure of a patent foramen ovale is associated with a decrease in prevalence of migraine. Neurology 2004;62(8): 1439–40.

36. Reisman M, Christofferson RD, Jesurum J, et al. Migraine headache relief after transcatheter closure of patent foramen ovale. J Am Coll Cardiol 2005; 45(4):493–5.

37. Azarbal B, Tobis J, Suh W, et al. Association of interatrial shunts and migraine headaches: impact of transcatheter closure. J Am Coll Cardiol 2005; 45(4):489–92.

38. Donti A, Giardini A, Salomone L, et al. Transcatheter patent foramen ovale closure using the Premere PFO occlusion system. Catheter Cardiovasc Interv 2006;68(5):736–40.

39. Anzola GP, Frisoni GB, Morandi E, et al. Shunt-associated migraine responds favorably to atrial septal repair: a case-control study. Stroke 2006;37(2): 430–4.

40. Kimmelstiel C, Gange C, Thaler D. Is patent foramen ovale closure effective in reducing migraine symptoms? A controlled study. Catheter Cardiovasc Interv 2007;69(5):740–6.

41. Papa M, Gaspardone A, Fragasso G, et al. Usefulness of transcatheter patent foramen ovale closure in migraineurs with moderate to large right-to-left shunt and instrumental evidence of cerebrovascular damage. Am J Cardiol 2009; 104(3):434–9.

Indications and Imaging Modality of Choice in Pediatric Headache

Asha Sarma, MD[a],*, Tina Young Poussaint, MD[b]

KEYWORDS

- Pediatrics • Headache • Neuroimaging • Magnetic resonance imaging • Decision support

KEY POINTS

- Neuroimaging is generally not indicated for primary pediatric headache (tension, migraine, and cluster headaches).
- Practice parameters, including the 2017 American College of Radiology Appropriateness Criteria, are available to guide neuroimaging in pediatric headache.
- CT and MR imaging are first-line modalities for pediatric headache evaluation. Optimization of CT and MR imaging may decrease ionizing radiation exposure and need for procedural anesthesia.

INTRODUCTION

Pediatric headache is common and is associated with significant morbidity and economic cost.[1] Despite the increasing use of neuroimaging, findings that change clinical or surgical management are unusual in the absence of neurologic abnormalities.[2-5]

A variety of benign and emergent conditions can cause pediatric headache. This review aims to help guide when to image a child with headache and how to select the appropriate examination. Optimization of CT and MR imaging evaluation with tailored, indication-based protocoling is considered in detail, along with approaches to imaging in a range of specific clinical conditions.

EPIDEMIOLOGY

The reported prevalence of pediatric headache ranges from approximately 17% to 91%.[6,7] Prevalence increases with age throughout childhood and adolescence but headaches are still common in young children—for instance, 29% of children under age 5 have reported a headache within the previous year.[6,8] Headaches are more prevalent in boys before puberty. This trend reverses after puberty, with the female-to-male ratio increasing into adulthood.[9]

PEDIATRIC HEADACHE CLASSIFICATION

Generally, uncomplicated primary headache disorders without an underlying cause (eg, migraine, tension, cluster, and daily headaches) do not require neuroimaging.[10] Causes of secondary headache are numerous and varied.

Headaches can also be classified as acute, acute recurrent (episodic), chronic nonprogressive, chronic progressive, or new persistent (**Fig. 1**).[9] Acute recurrent (episodic) and chronic nonprogressive headaches tend to represent benign causes of headache (ie, primary headache disorders), whereas new persistent and chronic progressive headaches are more concerning for significant intracranial pathology and, therefore,

Disclosures: None.
[a] Department of Radiology, Vanderbilt University Medical Center, Monroe Carell Jr. Children's Hospital, 2200 Children's Way, Suite 1421, Nashville, TN 37232-9700, USA; [b] Department of Radiology, Harvard Medical School, Boston Children's Hospital, 300 Longwood Avenue, Boston, MA 02130, USA
* Corresponding author.
E-mail address: asha.sarma@vumc.org

Neuroimag Clin N Am 29 (2019) 271–289
https://doi.org/10.1016/j.nic.2019.01.007

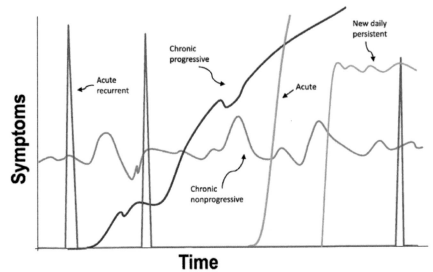

Fig. 1. Patterns of headache. (*From* Blume HK. Pediatric headache: a review. Pediatr Rev 2012;33(12):563; with permission.)

more often warrant neuroimaging.[9,11] Causes of acute single-event headaches range from self-limited viral upper respiratory infections to life-threatening hemorrhage from a vascular malformation—thus, these headaches must be carefully triaged.[9]

CLINICAL CONSIDERATIONS IN PEDIATRIC PATIENTS WITH HEADACHE
Clinical Evaluation of Pediatric Patients with Headache

Important components of the clinical evaluation for pediatric headache are included in **Table 1**.[9,12]

Knowledge of intracranial and head and neck pain–sensitive structures may help in lesion localization (**Table 2**).[13] Migraine-like pain is believed caused by cortical spreading depression, defined as sequential waves of neuronal depolarization and depressed neuronal activity, leading to release of chemicals that irritate trigeminal nerve afferents.[14]

Red Flags in Pediatric Patients with Headache

Research has been focused on determining clinical signs and symptoms predictive of serious intracranial pathology (red flags) in patients with headache.[1] Brain tumors are a common concern (although tumor is uncommon without neurologic signs).[4,15–17]

Dodick[18] established a set of red flags in pediatric patients with headache that fit the memorable mnemonic, SNOOPPPPY (**Box 1**). These red flags have not been rigorously validated in pediatric patients, and there is some disagreement in the literature about whether patients should be imaged on the basis of age at presentation, change in headache type, and occipital headache.[1] In a study of pediatric patients in the emergency setting, preschool age, recent onset of pain, occipital location, inability to describe the quality of pain, and objective neurologic signs predicted serious pathology.[19]

Summary of Current Clinical Guidelines for Neuroimaging Pediatric Patients with Headache

Relevant clinical guidelines for neuroimaging pediatric patients with headache are summarized in **Table 3**.[11,20,21]

IMAGING EVALUATION OF PEDIATRIC PATIENTS WITH HEADACHE
General Considerations

Noncontrast CT and MR imaging are the most commonly used modalities in the initial evaluation of pediatric headache. Clinical evaluation, resource availability (including anesthesia services), and risk-benefit analyses addressing radiation exposure and sedation influence choice of modality.

CT is generally more widely available than MR imaging in the pediatric emergency setting; however, efforts have been made to increase the availability of MR imaging due to concerns about carcinogenesis from ionizing radiation.[22,23] An advantage of CT over MR imaging is more rapid examination speed that reduces the need for sedation. CT is also more useful in clinically

Table 1
Salient components of the clinical evaluation of pediatric patients with headache

Headache Features	Past Medical History	Family History	Drugs and Medications	Social History	Physical and Neurologic Examination Findings	Ancillary Testing
Temporal pattern	Tumor predisposition syndromes	Migraine	Stimulants (eg, for attention-deficit hyperactivity disorder)	Social stressors	Significantly abnormal height and weight	Blood tests
Location	Sinus disease	Familial tumor syndromes	Bronchodilators	Sleep patterns	Abnormal vital signs (eg, fever, hypertension)	CSF opening pressure and analysis
Character	Cerebrovascular disease (eg, moyamoya, sickle cell disease)	Polycystic kidney disease, berry aneurysms	Drugs of abuse, including alcohol		Signs of external bleeding	Electroencephalogram
Triggers and warning signs	Bleeding disorder		Minocycline (can cause intracranial hypertension)		Altered mental status	
Red flag signs			Caffeine		Dysphasia	
					Altered motor or sensory function	
					Cranial nerve palsy	
					Abnormal vision	
					Abnormal gait	
					Papilledema, optic atrophy, intraocular hemorrhage	

Data from Refs.[10–12]

Table 2
Pain-sensitive structures of the brain, head, and neck

Intracranial Pain–sensitive Structures	Head and Neck Pain–sensitive Structures
Dural venous sinuses	Skin, pericranium,
Anterior and middle	subcutaneous tissues,
meningeal arteries,	muscles, extracranial
portions of the	arteries
internal carotid	C2 and C3 nerves
artery, and arterial	Eyes, ears, teeth,
branches near the	sinuses
circle of Willis	Oropharynx
Skull base dura	Nasal cavity mucosa
Cranial nerves V, IX,	
and X	
Periaqueductal gray	
matter	
Sensory nuclei of the	
thalami	

Data from Headache & facial pain. In: Aminoff MJ, Greenberg DA, Simon RP, editors. Clinical neurology, 9th edition. New York: McGraw-Hill; 2015.

unstable patients and in those with certain implanted devices (eg, pacemaker and cochlear implant devices).

MR imaging is generally more expensive, less available, and more time consuming than CT. It is the modality of choice, however, for the initial evaluation of most types of pediatric headache (excluding sudden-onset thunderclap headaches, which usually are first evaluated with CT) due to its superior tissue contrast resolution, which enables more optimal tissue characterization and

Box 1
SNOOPPPPY mnemonic for red flags in pediatric headache

S: systemic symptoms or illness

N: neurologic signs or symptoms

O: onset recent or sudden (ie, thunderclap headache)

O: occipital localization of pain

P: pattern—precipitated by Valsalva maneuver

P: pattern—positional

P: pattern—progressive

P: parents—no family history

Y: years—age less than 6

From Dodick D. Headache as a symptom of ominous disease. What are the warning signals? Postgrad Med 1997;101(5):46–50, 55-46, 62-44.

detection of small or subtle lesions. Furthermore, unlike CT, MR imaging uses electromagnetic radiation, which confers no carcinogenic risk.

Optimization of use of gadolinium-based contrast agents is essential for MR imaging. Recent studies have shown that gadolinium deposition occurs in the brain, bone, and other organs in children with normal renal function.[24–29] The physiologic and clinical significance of brain gadolinium deposition (if any) has not yet been determined; however, judicious use of gadolinium-based contrast agents is recommended.

For MR imaging, procedural sedation to minimize patient motion is often necessary to achieve diagnostic quality imaging. Although short (<3 hour), single sessions of sedation in otherwise healthy infants or children likely has no lasting neurodevelopmental consequences, studies of animals, including nonhuman primates, have raised concern about the safety of anesthetic agents in children.[30] Awareness of this issue increased after the US Food and Drug Administration issued warnings that anesthesia administered to children under age 3 for sessions longer than 3 hours or on a repeated basis might affect brain development.[31]

At Boston Children's Hospital, strategies for minimizing the need for anesthesia in children (**Box 2**) have substantially decreased the proportion of cases requiring anesthesia. Importantly, it may be unsafe to defer indicated neuroimaging studies in many instances, and sedation and general anesthesia remain vital tools.[30]

Specific CT and MR Imaging Protocol Considerations

Noncontrast MR imaging is the study of choice for most pediatric patients with headache (**Box 3**). Susceptibility-weighted imaging (SWI); MR arteriography or MR venography; perfusion sequences, such as arterial spin labeling (ASL); isotropic 3-D fast turbo spin-echo sequences; postcontrast sequences; and MR spectroscopy may be added for evaluation of specific disorders.

Using conventional acquisition parameters, headache evaluation currently requires approximately 45 minutes to an hour to complete at Boston Children's Hospital. *Fast brain*, or rapidly acquired, sequences can be performed on 3T MR imaging units to decrease acquisition time and reduce the need for anesthesia.[32] Generally, these are commercially available sequences that are modified using parallel imaging with higher

Table 3
Summary of relevant clinical guidelines for neuroimaging in pediatric headache

2002 American Academy of Neurology and Child Neurology Society

No neuroimaging in children with recurrent headaches and a normal neurologic examination

Imaging should be considered with abnormal neurologic examination, recent onset of severe headache, change in headache type, evidence of neurologic dysfunction

2013 Choosing Wisely campaign (American Board of Internal Medicine and American Headache Society)

Neuroimaging not recommended with stable migraine headaches

MR imaging (when available) preferred over CT in the nonemergent evaluation of headache

2017 American College of Radiology Appropriateness Criteria for Headache–Child[11]

Type of headache (initial imaging)	Appropriate imaging modality or modalities (usually appropriate in italics)
Primary headache	Imaging usually not appropriate
Secondary headache	*MR imaging without or without and with contrast* MR imaging with MR arteriography or MR venography CT without or with contrast
Headache due to remote trauma	*MR imaging without contrast*
Headache attributed to infection	*MR imaging without and with contrast* MR imaging without contrast MR imaging with MR arteriography or MR venography CT without or with contrast
Thunderclap headache	*CT without contrast* *MR arteriography without contrast* *MR imaging without contrast* CTA

Data from Refs.[11,20,21]

acceleration factors, gradient echo T1-weighted imaging, and elimination of manual intersequence adjustments.[32] At Boston Children's Hospital, typical fast brain MR imaging studies are currently approximately 11 minutes in duration. Fast brain sequences are often useful in headache patients who are approximately 4 years to 7 years of age and in many older children and adolescents, including those with developmental delay. Diagnostic quality can be comparable to standard acquisitions.[32] On 1.5T MR imaging units, periodically rotated overlapping parallel lines with enhanced reconstruction imaging is sometimes used to decrease scan times. At Boston Children's Hospital, rapid axial T2-weighted echo-planar fast spin-echo imaging is often used to rapidly evaluate ventricular size in hydrocephalus patients with headache.[33]

CT may be used instead of MR imaging in emergency and critical care settings, in patients with contraindications to MR imaging, and for evaluation of new focal neurologic deficits when MR imaging is less available. Strategies to reduce

Box 2
Strategies for minimizing anesthesia in neuroimaging

Real-time case monitoring with close communication between radiologists and technologists

Feed and swaddle technique (infants)

Dual-source CT

Fast brain MR imaging sequences on 3T units

Distraction techniques (eg, video goggles)

Patient selection and real-time intervention by child life specialists

Box 3
Basic MR imaging protocol for imaging of pediatric patients with headache

Sagittal T1-weighted 3D T1-weighted gradient echo sequence, reformatted into axial and coronal planes

Axial T2-weighted sequence

Axial fat-suppressed FLAIR sequence

Axial DTI

Coronal T2-weighted sequence

radiation dose in pediatric CT include patient weight/size–based parameter adjustments and selection of lower-dose parameters when higher image noise can be tolerated (eg, sinus disease, known hydrocephalus, and bone lesions). Dual-source CT can both decrease dose and decrease scan time to less than 1 second and, hence, decrease the need for sedation.

APPROACH TO IMAGING FOR PEDIATRIC HEADACHES CAUSED BY SPECIFIC CONDITIONS

Numerous underlying conditions can cause headaches in pediatric patients. This discussion briefly describes each entity, summarizing the epidemiology, clinical presentation, optimal imaging study and protocol selection, and imaging findings. Table 4 lists adjunct sequences that may be added to routine MR imaging protocols for specific conditions.

Emergent Causes of Pediatric Headache

Hydrocephalus

Hydrocephalus is due to imbalance between production and absorption of cerebrospinal fluid (CSF) (Fig. 2) and is a rare cause of pediatric headache (<1%).[19,34] Early morning headache with nausea and vomiting, sometimes with changes in personality and behavior, is typical and may be accompanied by signs of elevated intracranial pressure.[35] Intracranial hemorrhage (ICH) or infection, aqueductal stenosis, Chiari malformations, and tumors are common causes.

Either CT or MR imaging may be appropriate for imaging evaluation. Radiographic shunt series are an important adjunct study.

Infection

Infection causing pediatric headaches can be broadly divided into systemic infection (eg, upper respiratory infection and febrile illnesses), head and neck infection (Fig. 3) (eg, sinusitis, otomastoiditis, and orbital infection), and primary central nervous system (CNS) infection (eg, meningitis, encephalitis, and abscess). Immunocompromised patients are at increased risk.

Head and neck and systemic infections are common, and sinus, mastoid, and middle ear mucosal disease and effusion are often incidentally detected even in asymptomatic pediatric patients.[36] Upper respiratory infection has been found to represent the most common cause of headache, in approximately 31% of patients.[19] It can be difficult to determine whether non-CNS systemic or head and neck infection is causal or merely concurrent with primary or other causes of secondary headache.[36] These infections are generally determined to be causal if headache symptoms parallel the course of the infection, headaches are typical for the type of infection, and infection has been clinically diagnosed.[10]

Primary CNS infections are much more rare (approximately 2% of cases presenting to the pediatric emergency department) and tend to present with systemic symptoms and laboratory abnormalities, meningismus, and neurologic signs or altered mental status.[10,19]

In suspected primary CNS infection, clinical and laboratory evaluations are essential. Headache, high fever, altered mental status, focal neurologic signs, and seizures may be indications for neuroimaging.[11] Noncontrast CT may be obtained prior to lumbar puncture when there is concern for intracranial mass effect or herniation.[11] MR imaging without and with contrast is the neuroimaging study of choice. MR imaging may help to distinguish infection from other clinical entities, detect complications (eg, meningitis, encephalitis, and intracranial abscess or empyema), and identify the causal pathogen.

Imaging is usually not indicated in acute uncomplicated sinusitis. Noncontrast CT is indicated for persistent sinusitis. Noncontrast CT or MR imaging without and with contrast are indicated when there is concern for orbital or intracranial complications.[11]

Tumor

Brain tumors are a *do-not-miss* diagnosis and a common cause of concern among patients, parents, and referring providers (Fig. 4). Headache is a common early symptom and presenting complaint (particularly for posterior fossa tumors), found in 62% to 88% of cases.[16] Tumors are usually accompanied, however, by neurologic signs and are found in fewer than 1% of children with isolated headaches.[16,34]

CT is often performed in the emergent setting, especially for assessment of significant mass effect, hemorrhage, acute hydrocephalus, or herniation. MR imaging performed without and with contrast is superior for presurgical evaluation, including assessment of disease extent. Advanced imaging techniques, such as diffusion-weighted imaging (DWI), perfusion imaging, and MR spectroscopy, can provide physiologic evaluation of tumors.

Brain ischemia

Headaches are a common presenting feature of ischemic stroke in children, found in

Table 4
Summary of suggested adjunct MR imaging sequences for tailoring imaging assessment in specific conditions

Condition	Sequences
Hydrocephalus	T2 echo-planar fast spin-echo (*ventricle check* MR imaging) Sagittal T2-weighted fast spin-echo sequence to determine endoscopic third ventriculostomy patency
Primary CNS infection	Postgadolinium T1-weighted sequence SWI (septic emboli, hemorrhagic infection [eg, herpes encephalitis]) MR arteriography, MR venography (vasospasm, CSVT)
Head and neck infection	Postgadolinium T1-weighted gradient-echo sequence Postgadolinium fat-suppressed T1-weighted sequence (2 planes) Fat-suppressed T2-weighted sequence (2 planes) MR venography
Brain tumor	SWI MR spectroscopy ASL and/or dynamic contrast-enhanced perfusion imaging Postgadolinium T1-weighted spine imaging (assessment for CSF dissemination) MR arteriography, MR venography
Stroke	SWI ASL MR arteriography MR venography Postgadolinium T1-weighted sequence
ICH due to an underlying tumor or vascular lesion	SWI MR arteriography Postgadolinium 3D T1-weighted spin-echo (tumor) and/or gradient echo (vascular lesion) sequences
Hemiplegic migraine	SWI ASL MR arteriography
Vasculopathy (eg, PACNS, moyamoya)	SWI MR arteriography ASL, velocity selective-ASL Vessel wall imaging
CSVT	MR venography Postgadolinium 3D T1-weighted gradient echo sequence
PRES	SWI ASL MR arteriography
Chiari I malformation	T2-weighted sagittal and axial sequences of the cervical spine Phase contrast or cine sequence CSF flow study Spinal cord DTI sequence
Non-neoplastic cysts	T2-weighted balanced steady-state gradient echo sequence T2-weighted echo-planar fast spin-echo sequence Sagittal T2-weighted spin-echo sequence (pineal region lesions causing aqueductal obstruction)
Mitochondrial disease	SWI MR spectroscopy
Idiopathic intracranial hypertension	MR venography Postgadolinium 3D T1-weighted gradient echo sequence (vascular imaging is to exclude CSVT)

approximately a quarter to half of affected children, usually with accompanying focal neurologic deficits.[37,38] Headache may be a more common stroke symptom in children than in adults.[37,38] Arterial ischemia-related headaches are more common in children over 5 years of age (possibly due to greater ability to verbalize symptoms), with increasing incidence

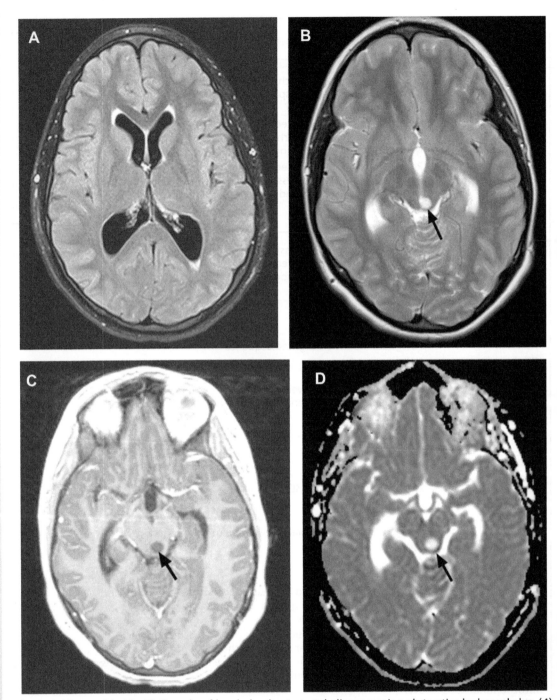

Fig. 2. A 12-year-old girl with 2 weeks of headache due to tectal glioma causing obstructive hydrocephalus. (A) Axial FLAIR MR imaging demonstrates mildly dilated lateral ventricles with transependymal edema. Axial T2-weighted (B) and postgadolinium 3D T1-weighted gradient echo images (C) and apparent diffusion coefficient map (D) demonstrate a nonenhancing small, round tectal tumor with T2 prolongation and facilitated diffusion (arrows). The patient underwent endoscopic third ventriculostomy.

into adolescence. Headaches are more common in vascular dissection and transient arteriopathy of childhood (approximately 70% each).[37]

CT is often the first study chosen in the emergency setting and is used to evaluate for hemorrhage or large territorial infarction (contraindications to thrombolysis).[39,40] MR imaging is more

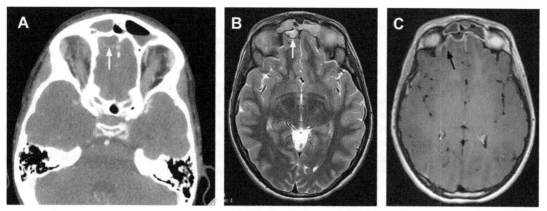

Fig. 3. A 15-year-old boy with 4 days of headache, fever, and eye swelling due to acute, complicated sinusitis. Axial CT with contrast (*A*) and axial T2-weighted MR imaging (*B*) demonstrate frontal sinus opacification with air-fluid levels and a small right frontal epidural abscess (*arrows*). Postgadolinium 3D T1-weighted spin-echo sequence (*C*) shows leptomeningeal enhancement adjacent to the abscess (*arrow*), concerning for meningitis.

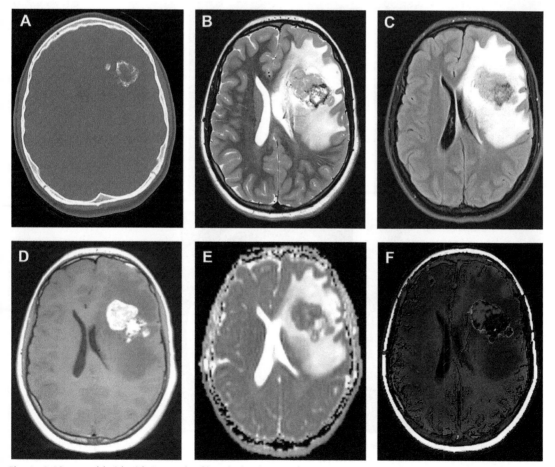

Fig. 4. A 16-year-old girl with 1 month of headache due to a brain tumor. Axial CT (*A*) and T2-weighted (*B*), FLAIR (*C*), postgadolinium 3D T1-weighted spin-echo (*D*), apparent diffusion coefficient map (*E*), and post-processed dynamic contrast-enhanced perfusion (*F*) MR images show a partially calcified, enhancing intra-axial tumor with low diffusivity, elevated blood flow, extensive surrounding vasogenic edema, and mild mass effect. The resected lesion represented anaplastic ganglioglioma.

sensitive for acute ischemia. CT and MR imaging findings vary with timing relative to the ischemic insult.

Intracranial hemorrhage due to underlying vascular lesions

Nontraumatic acute ICH in pediatric patients is often caused by underlying vascular lesions (eg, arteriovenous malformations [AVMs] [Fig. 5], aneurysms, and cavernous malformations). Noncontrast CT is usually the initial study for evaluation of pediatric patients with thunderclap headache and suspected acute ICH.

Headache is relatively common in patients with AVM even without ICH, with a wide range of reported incidence of 9% to 70% of cases at presentation.[41] Headaches commonly localize to the side of the lesion. Occipital location is a risk factor for headache, which is often associated with visual symptoms.[41]

Less than 5% of intracranial arterial aneurysms present in children. Most affect children older than 5 years of age, and aneurysms are approximately twice as common in boys.[42] They are more commonly found at the internal carotid artery bifurcation and in the posterior circulation than in adults, and mycotic, giant, and posttraumatic aneurysms are more common.[42] Headache is a common presenting symptom, affecting 82% of patients, with a median 2-week prodrome.[42] Seizure and cranial neuropathies are more common in children than in adults.[42]

CMs are vascular malformations comprised of dilated endothelium-lined blood vessels without

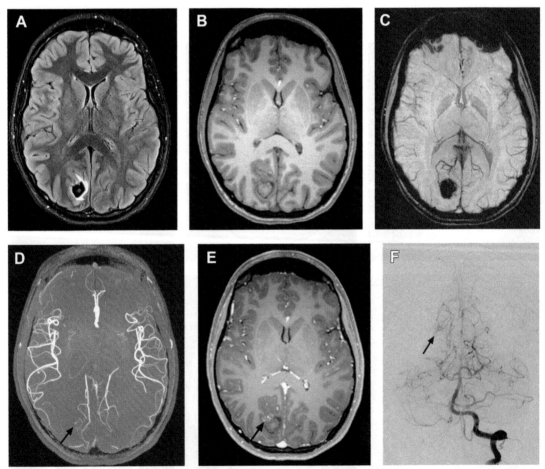

Fig. 5. A 15-year-old girl with headache and visual field cut due to an AVM-related hemorrhage. Axial FLAIR (A), 3D T1-weighted gradient echo (B), and SWI (C) MR images demonstrate a small right occipital hematoma with mild surrounding vasogenic edema. Axial time-of-flight MR arteriography maximum intensity projection image (D) and postgadolinium 3D T1-weighted gradient echo (E) demonstrate a small vascular nidus (arrows). (F) Left vertebral artery injection image from a conventional angiogram obtained several months later, after resolution of the hematoma, demonstrates the nidus (arrow). The nidus was angiographically occult at presentation due to compression of the small vessels by the hematoma. The AVM was resected.

muscular and adventitial layers.[43,44] Approximately one-quarter present in pediatric patients.[43] In children under 6 years old, lesions tend to be larger and are more likely to bleed than in children over 12 years old. At presentation, headaches (approximately 3%) are less common than seizures (38%), focal neurologic deficits (42%), and intracranial hypertension (29%).[43]

For evaluation of underlying vascular lesions, CT arteriography and MR imaging, including precontrast and postcontrast vascular imaging, may be complementary. Soft tissue contrast resolution of CTA is lower than that of MR imaging, but its higher spatial resolution and decreased sensitivity to motion artifact can be helpful in detecting abnormal vessels. If no underlying lesion is found, conventional angiography and/or delayed follow-up imaging after resolution of any hematoma that may be compressing abnormal vessels or obscuring tumor (usually weeks to months after the acute hemorrhage) is indicated. Conventional contrast angiography is also used for image-guided intervention.

Vascular Causes of Headache Without Acute Hemorrhage

Hemiplegic migraine

Hemiplegic migraine is a rare migraine variant (approximately 4% in 1 large pediatric series)[45] that mimics cerebral infarction (**Fig. 6**).[10,45] Migraine with aura is accompanied by fully reversible motor, visual, sensory, and/or speech and language deficits that usually last less than 72 hours but may persist for weeks.[10] Familial cases are often caused by membrane channel mutations (eg, CACNA1A, ATP1A2, and SCN1A).[46]

MR imaging may be normal during an acute episode or include findings of unilateral cortical swelling and hyperintensity on fluid-attenuated

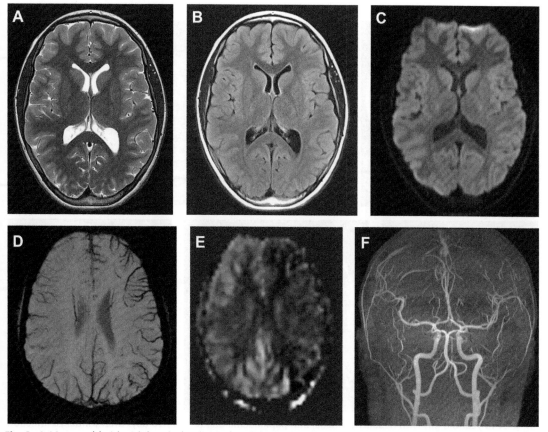

Fig. 6. A 14-year-old girl with headache due to hemiplegic migraine, presenting with transient aphasia and right-sided weakness. Axial T2-weighted (*A*), FLAIR (*B*), and DWI (*C*) MR images are normal. Axial SWI (*D*) demonstrates asymmetric venous prominence in the left cerebral hemisphere, suggesting increased tissue oxygen extraction. ASL (*E*) shows decreased flow in the left cerebral hemisphere, and coronal maximum intensity projection 3-D reconstruction from time-of-flight MR arteriography (*F*) shows pruning of distal left middle cerebral artery branches. Imaging abnormalities resolved on 3-week follow-up MR imaging (not pictured).

inversion recovery (FLAIR) and T2-weighted imaging, decreased perfusion, diminished caliber of vessels on MR arteriography, and asymmetric prominence of cortical veins on SWI due to increased tissue oxygen extraction and elevated venous deoxyhemoglobin. Normal DWI excludes ischemic injury. Imaging abnormalities resolve on follow-up.[46–48] Transient neurologic deficits with similar imaging findings can be seen even without migraine in an entity that has been termed *regional cerebral hypoperfusion.*[49]

Vasculitis

In childhood primary angiitis of the CNS (PACNS), clinical and imaging features vary by type (nonprogressive, progressive, and small-vessel angiography-negative, biopsy-positive types).[50] Serum inflammatory markers are typically elevated.[51] Ischemia-induced headache accompanied by focal neurologic deficits or seizures is common in angiography-positive disease.[50]

MR imaging is the imaging modality of choice. Time-of-flight MR arteriography may overestimate or underestimate abnormalities.[50] ICH may affect decisions pertaining to thrombolysis. Perfusion imaging is helpful for evaluating tissue at risk. CTA may be useful to evaluate MR arteriography abnormalities that are suspected to represent artifact, whereas conventional angiography is the gold standard for evaluation of the vessels.[50,51] Using postgadolinium T1-weighted spin-echo imaging at 3T, thickening and increased enhancement of the vessel wall may be detected even in nonstenotic arteries.[52]

Cerebral sinovenous thrombosis

Cerebral sinovenous thrombosis (CSVT) is rare in children (**Fig. 7**).[53] Although seizures are the most common presenting clinical feature overall (a majority of cases are in neonates and infants under 6 months), older children typically present with headaches (32%–68%) and motor symptoms.[53,54]

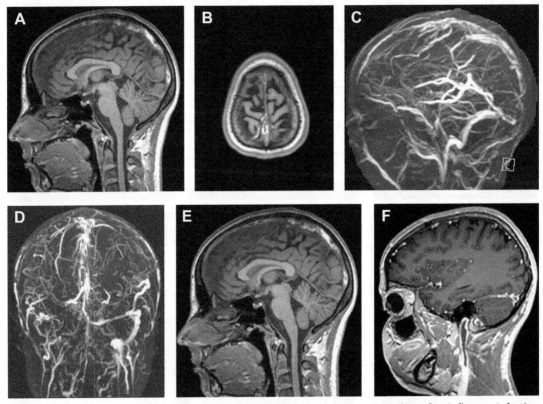

Fig. 7. A 16-year-old girl with headache, ataxia, and papilledema due to CSVT 10 days after influenza infection. Sagittal and axial 3D T1-weighted gradient echo MR images (*A, B*) demonstrate extensive hyperintense thrombus within the superior sagittal sinus and tributary cortical veins. Sagittal and coronal maximum intensity projection 3-D reconstructions from time-of-flight MR venography (*C, D*) demonstrate loss of flow-related enhancement within the superior sagittal sinus and right transverse and sigmoid sinuses and upper internal jugular vein. Postcontrast sagittal 3D T1-weighted gradient echo (*E, F*) demonstrates filling defects in the same distribution. MR imaging showed findings of elevated intracranial pressure (not pictured).

Complications may include hemorrhagic infarction (40%) and hydrocephalus.[54]

When CSVT is suspected, CT venography or MR venography is indicated even if initial CT is normal. On noncontrast CT, involved veins may appear hyperdense (>70 Hounsfield units) and distended. Absent flow-related enhancement on MR venography may correspond to intravenous filling defects on CT venography and postcontrast 3D T1-weighted gradient echo imaging.[54] Involvement of multiple veins is common (70%).[53] MR imaging can evaluate for edema, ischemia, and hemorrhagic infarction with high sensitivity and specificity.[54]

Posterior reversible encephalopathy syndrome
Posterior reversible encephalopathy syndrome (PRES) results from failed cerebrovascular autoregulation or cytotoxic endothelial injury. Risk factors include renal or autoimmune disease, malignancy, hypertension (85%), and chemotherapy or immunosuppressive therapy. Seizure (90%), encephalopathy, headache (40%), and visual disturbances are common in pediatric patients.

CT is often the initial imaging modality for suspected PRES; however, MR imaging should be obtained even when CT is normal. Findings on CT and MR can include hemispheric edema. In typical PRES, this most often presents in the parietal and occipital lobes, followed by the frontal lobes and cerebellum.[55] Atypical PRES is more common in children than adults, with relatively greater involvement of the frontal and temporal lobes and deep gray matter.[56] More frequent involvement of the cerebellum has not been universal across studies.[57] Low diffusivity and hemorrhage are overall less common atypical features that may be more frequent in children.[56] Perfusion sequences may show regional hypoperfusion and hyperperfusion, and angiographic imaging may show diffuse arterial constriction, narrowing, and beading.[58]

Moyamoya vasculopathy
Moyamoya vasculopathy is characterized by progressive steno-occlusive disease of the internal carotid artery and its terminal branches, with resultant formation of puff-of-smoke lenticulostriate and leptomeningeal collaterals (Fig. 8). Headaches are common before and after revascularization surgery and may resemble migraines, although may be refractory to usual pharmacologic therapy. Headaches may be caused by hypoperfusion or redistributed blood flow.[59]

Although conventional angiography is usually necessary to define disease extent, MR imaging with MR arteriography plays an important role at diagnosis and in follow-up for assessment of sulcal bright signal on FLAIR (ivy sign), infarction, vascular steno-occlusive disease, and collateral vessels. ASL may show regions of decreased flow due to increased path length of labeled spins through leptomeningeal collateral vessels; velocity selective ASL (vs-ASL) may reflect perfusion more accurately.[60]

Chiari I Malformation

Chiari I malformation is defined by cerebellar tonsillar descent to at least 5 mm below the foramen magnum. Headache is the most common presenting symptom, with Chiari I malformation identified in approximately 6% of children imaged for headache and 12% with the malformation presenting with headache (Fig. 9).[61,62] Chiari I malformation frequently coexists with primary headache and many patients meeting imaging criteria are asymptomatic; therefore, clinical correlation is required. Specific clinical features linking headaches to Chiari I malformation include occipital location; precipitation by Valsalva maneuver; short duration; and bulbar, cerebellar, lower cranial nerve, and upper cervical spinal cord signs.[10] Greater tonsillar descent is associated with greater headache severity.[63] Occipital headaches and those that are precipitated by Valsalva-like maneuvers are more likely to respond to surgical intervention.[10]

Advanced MR imaging sequences, such as cardiac-gated phase contrast for CSF flow assessment, pulse-gated cine for cerebellar tonsillar motion, quantitative volumetric assessment of the posterior fossa and biometry of the skull base, and spinal cord diffusion tensor imaging (DTI), have been investigated but are not currently in wide clinical use.[64]

Non-neoplastic Cysts and Their Complications

Arachnoid cyst
Arachnoid cysts form when CSF accumulates between the walls of a duplicated arachnoid membrane (Fig. 10). Most are found in children and young adults, commonly as an incidental finding.[61,65] Incidence in pediatric patients with headache is approximately 1% to 3%.[61] Rare complications include enlarging cyst (children under 4 years of age), intracystic and subdural hemorrhage (especially after trauma), and obstructive hydrocephalus.[65,66]

MR imaging assessment may include a balanced steady-state gradient echo sequence for delineation of the cyst wall. At Boston

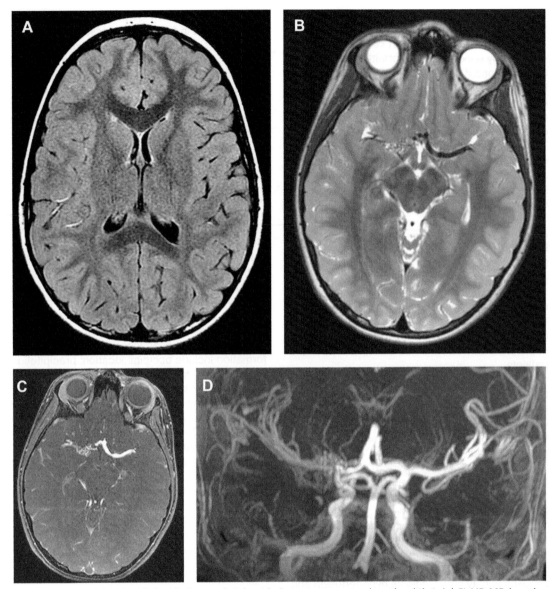

Fig. 8. A 9-year-old girl with headaches and right-sided moyamoya vasculopathy. (*A*) Axial FLAIR MR imaging demonstrates ivy sign connoting leptomeningeal collateral flow in the right cerebral hemisphere. Axial T2-weighted image (*B*), axial time-of-flight MR arteriography image (*C*), and coronal time-of-flight MR arteriography maximum intensity projection 3-D reconstruction (*D*) demonstrate severe narrowing of the right internal carotid artery terminus and the A1 and M1 segments, with numerous middle cerebral artery (MCA) cistern collaterals and pruning of distal MCA branches. The patient was treated with pial synangiosis.

Children's Hospital, echo-planar fast spin-echo imaging often is used to follow arachnoid cysts for changes in size or fluid reaccumulation after surgery.

Colloid cyst

Colloid cysts, believed to arise from endodermal remnants at the roof of the embryonic diencephalon, are rare in children, with fewer than 8% presenting before 15 years of age.[65]

Approximately 50% to 60% of symptomatic patients have headaches, often with papilledema. Precipitous frontal headaches and nausea and vomiting that are relieved when the patient is lying down are characteristic.[65] Acute hydrocephalus may result in sudden neurologic deterioration or death. Noncontrast CT and/or MR imaging demonstrate a round lesion at the roof of the third ventricle near the foramen of Monro, which is hyperdense

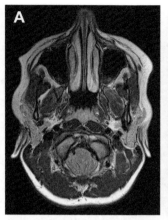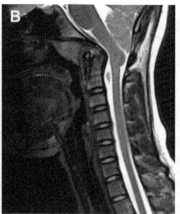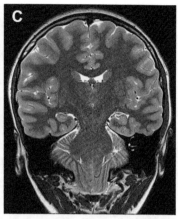

Fig. 9. A 13-year-old girl with brief headaches and syncopal episodes due to Chiari I malformation. Axial, sagittal, and coronal T2-weighted MR images (*A–C*) show cerebellar tonsillar descent below the foramen magnum, with crowding of the adjacent CSF spaces and dorsal bump at the cervicomedullary junction. The patient underwent posterior fossa decompression.

on CT, with variable signal intensity on MR imaging.[65]

Miscellaneous Conditions

Mitochondrial disease
Migraine-like headaches that have been attributed to vasculopathy are common in mitochondrial encephalopathy with lactic acidosis and stroke-like episodes (MELAS).[10] Both tension-type and migraine-like headaches, however, are common even in mitochondrial disorders without vasculopathy, suggesting pathogenesis related to abnormal mitochondrial metabolism.[67]

In MELAS, neuroimaging findings include stroke-like lesions crossing vascular territories;

deep gray matter changes including basal ganglia mineralization; white matter abnormalities and parenchymal volume loss; and elevated lactate in the parenchyma and CSF on MR spectroscopy.[68]

Idiopathic intracranial hypertension
Idiopathic intracranial hypertension is rare in children, in particular those under 10 years of age, with most cases of intracranial hypertension being secondary (**Fig. 11**). The predilection for female and obese patients that has been described in adults has not been observed in pediatric patients. Headache is the most common symptom, occurring in greater than 90% of affected patients.[69]

Hartmann and colleagues[70] found no significant difference between children and adults in MR

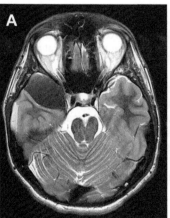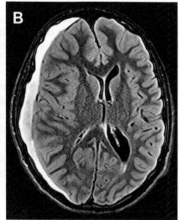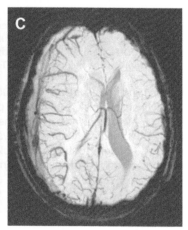

Fig. 10. A 17-year-old boy with 2 months of headache, presenting with worsening headache and vomiting due to hemorrhage complicating an arachnoid cyst. Axial T2-weighted MR image (*A*) demonstrates a right middle cranial fossa arachnoid cyst containing hypointense blood products. Axial FLAIR (*B*) and SWI (*C*) demonstrate a right holohemispheric subdural hematoma with mass effect and venous congestion in the right cerebral hemisphere.

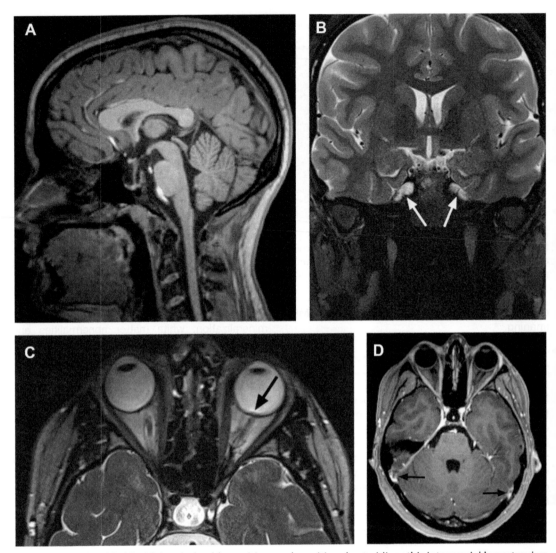

Fig. 11. A 17-year-old girl with headache, blurry vision, and vomiting due to idiopathic intracranial hypertension. Sagittal 3D T1-weighted gradient echo image (*A*) demonstrates a partially empty sella. Coronal T2-weighted MR image (*B*) demonstrates enlarged Meckel caves (*arrows*). Axial T2-weighted MR image (*C*) demonstrates flattening of the posterior globes and subtle elevation of the left optic papilla (*arrow*). Axial postgadolinium T1-weighted 3D T1-weighted gradient echo (*D*) shows flattening of the transverse sinuses at the sinodural angle (*arrows*). There was no evidence of CSVT.

imaging findings of optic nerve tortuosity and optic nerve head protrusion, increased perioptic CSF, tonsillar herniation, and enlargement of Meckel cave. Optic nerve enhancement was more common in prepubertal patients, and scleral flattening, transverse sinus stenosis, meningoceles, and sellar changes were less common.

SUMMARY

Pediatric headache is a common clinical problem and reason for neuroimaging referral. The yield of imaging is low in patients with primary headache disorders. There are many secondary causes of pediatric headache, for which neuroimaging tends to be more useful. Multiple published clinical guidelines are available to guide imaging modality selection. Tailored CT and MR selection and protocoling are key for optimal use and should include incorporation of shortened examinations, which decrease the need for anesthesia in pediatric neuroimaging.

REFERENCES

1. Trofimova A, Vey BL, Mullins ME, et al. Imaging of children with nontraumatic headaches. AJR Am J Roentgenol 2018;210(1):8–17.

2. Gilbert JW, Johnson KM, Larkin GL, et al. Atraumatic headache in US emergency departments: recent trends in CT/MRI utilisation and factors associated with severe intracranial pathology. Emerg Med J 2012;29(7):576–81.

3. Larson DB, Johnson LW, Schnell BM, et al. Rising use of CT in child visits to the emergency department in the United States, 1995-2008. Radiology 2011;259(3):793–801.

4. Rho YI, Chung HJ, Suh ES, et al. The role of neuro-imaging in children and adolescents with recurrent headaches–multicenter study. Headache 2011; 51(3):403–8.

5. Abu-Arafeh I, Macleod S. Serious neurological disorders in children with chronic headache. Arch Dis Child 2005;90(9):937–40.

6. Lateef TM, Merikangas KR, He J, et al. Headache in a national sample of American children: prevalence and comorbidity. J Child Neurol 2009;24(5): 536–43.

7. Abu-Arafeh I, Razak S, Sivaraman B, et al. Prevalence of headache and migraine in children and adolescents: a systematic review of population-based studies. Dev Med child Neurol 2010;52(12): 1088–97.

8. Scheller JM. The history, epidemiology, and classification of headaches in childhood. Semin Pediatr Neurol 1995;2(2):102–8.

9. Blume HK. Pediatric headache: a review. Pediatr Rev 2012;33(12):562–76.

10. Headache Classification Committee of the International Headache Society (IHS) The International Classification of Headache Disorders, 3rd edition. Cephalalgia 2018;38(1):1–211.

11. Hayes LL, Palasis S, Bartel TT, et al. ACR appropriateness criteria® headache-child 2017. Available at: https://acsearch.acr.org/docs/69439/Narrative/. Accessed February 23, 2018.

12. Rothner AD. The evaluation of headaches in children and adolescents. Semin Pediatr Neurol 1995;2(2): 109–18.

13. Aminoff MJ, Greenberg DA, Simon RP. Headache & facial pain. Clinical neurology. 9th edition. New York: McGraw-Hill; 2015. Available at: https:// accessmedicine.mhmedical.com/content.aspx? bookid=1194&sectionid=78427211. Accessed July 23, 2018.

14. Borsook D, Maleki N, Burstein R. Migraine. In: Zigmond MJ, Coyle JT, editors. Neurobiology of brain disorders: biological basis of neurological and psychiatric disorders. 1st edition. Cambridge (MA): Academic Press; 2015. p. 693–708.

15. DeVries A, Young PC, Wall E, et al. CT scan utilization patterns in pediatric patients with recurrent headache. Pediatrics 2013;132(1):e1–8.

16. The epidemiology of headache among children with brain tumor. Headache in children with brain tumors. The Childhood Brain Tumor Consortium. J Neurooncol 1991;10(1):31–46.

17. Ahmed MA, Martinez A, Cahill D, et al. When to image neurologically normal children with headaches: development of a decision rule. Acta Paediatr 2010; 99(6):940–3.

18. Dodick D. Headache as a symptom of ominous disease. What are the warning signals? Postgrad Med 1997;101(5):46–50, 55-46, 62-44.

19. Conicella E, Raucci U, Vanacore N, et al. The child with headache in a pediatric emergency department. Headache 2008;48(7):1005–11.

20. Lewis DW, Ashwal S, Dahl G, et al. Practice parameter: evaluation of children and adolescents with recurrent headaches: report of the Quality Standards Subcommittee of the American Academy of Neurology and the Practice Committee of the Child Neurology Society. Neurology 2002;59(4):490–8.

21. Loder E, Weizenbaum E, Frishberg B, et al. Choosing wisely in headache medicine: the American Headache Society's list of five things physicians and patients should question. Headache 2013; 53(10):1651–9.

22. Goske MJ, Applegate KE, Boylan J, et al. The Image Gently campaign: working together to change practice. AJR Am J Roentgenol 2008;190(2):273–4.

23. Scheinfeld MH, Moon JY, Fagan MJ, et al. MRI usage in a pediatric emergency department: an analysis of usage and usage trends over 5 years. Pediatr Radiol 2017;47(3):327–32.

24. McDonald JS, McDonald RJ, Jentoft ME, et al. Intracranial gadolinium deposition following gadodiamide-enhanced magnetic resonance imaging in pediatric patients: a case-control study. JAMA Pediatr 2017;171(7):705–7.

25. McDonald RJ, McDonald JS, Kallmes DF, et al. Intracranial gadolinium deposition after contrast-enhanced MR imaging. Radiology 2015;275(3): 772–82.

26. McDonald RJ, McDonald JS, Kallmes DF, et al. Gadolinium deposition in human brain tissues after contrast-enhanced MR imaging in adult patients without intracranial abnormalities. Radiology 2017; 285(2):546–54.

27. Radbruch A, Haase R, Kieslich PJ, et al. No signal intensity increase in the dentate nucleus on unenhanced T1-weighted MR images after more than 20 serial injections of macrocyclic gadolinium-based contrast agents. Radiology 2017;282(3): 699–707.

28. McDonald RJ, McDonald JS, Dai D, et al. Comparison of gadolinium concentrations within multiple rat organs after intravenous administration of linear versus macrocyclic gadolinium chelates. Radiology 2017;285(2):536–45.

29. Lord ML, Chettle DR, Grafe JL, et al. Observed deposition of gadolinium in bone using a new

noninvasive in vivo biomedical device: results of a small pilot feasibility study. Radiology 2018;287(1):96–103.

30. Andropoulos DB, Greene MF. Anesthesia and developing brains - implications of the FDA warning. N Engl J Med 2017;376(10):905–7.

31. FDA Drug Safety Communication: FDA approves label changes for use of general anesthetic and sedation drugs in young children. In: US Food and Drug Administration. 2017. Available at: https://www.fda.gov/Drugs/DrugSafety/ucm554634.htm. Accessed March 23, 2018.

32. Prakkamakul S, Witzel T, Huang S, et al. Ultrafast brain MRI: clinical deployment and comparison to conventional brain MRI at 3T. J Neuroimaging 2016;26(5):503–10.

33. Robson CD, MacDougall RD, Madsen JR, et al. Neuroimaging of children with surgically treated hydrocephalus: a practical approach. AJR Am J Roentgenol 2017;208(2):413–9.

34. Yilmaz U, Celegen M, Yilmaz TS, et al. Childhood headaches and brain magnetic resonance imaging findings. Eur J Paediatr Neurol 2014;18(2):163–70.

35. Ahad R, Kossoff EH. Secondary intracranial causes for headaches in children. Curr Pain Headache Rep 2008;12(5):373–8.

36. Vieira Neto RJ, Teixeira KCS, Guerreiro MM, et al. Paranasal sinus disease in children with headache. J Child Neurol 2017;32(12):1014–7.

37. Headache far more common stroke symptom in children than adults. In: American Heart Association/American Stroke Association Newsroom. 2017. Available at: http://newsroom.heart.org/news/headache-far-more-common-stroke-symptom-in-children-than-adults. Accessed April 3, 2018.

38. Mallick AA, Ganesan V, Kirkham FJ, et al. Childhood arterial ischaemic stroke incidence, presenting features, and risk factors: a prospective population-based study. Lancet Neurol 2014;13(1):35–43.

39. Rivkin MJ, deVeber G, Ichord RN, et al. Thrombolysis in pediatric stroke study. Stroke 2015;46(3):880–5.

40. Salmela MB, Mortazavi S, Jagadeesan BD, et al. ACR appropriateness criteria((R)) cerebrovascular disease. J Am Coll Radiol 2017;14(5S):S34–61.

41. Ellis JA, Mejia Munne JC, Lavine SD, et al. Arteriovenous malformations and headache. J Clin Neurosci 2016;23:38–43.

42. Garg K, Singh PK, Sharma BS, et al. Pediatric intracranial aneurysms–our experience and review of literature. Childs Nerv Syst 2014;30(5):873–83.

43. Bilginer B, Narin F, Hanalioglu S, et al. Cavernous malformations of the central nervous system (CNS) in children: clinico-radiological features and management outcomes of 36 cases. Childs Nerv Syst 2014;30(8):1355–66.

44. Osborn AG. Vascular malformations. In: Osborn AG, Hedlund GL, Salzman KL, editors. Osborn's brain: imaging, pathology, and anatomy. 2nd edition. Philadelphia: Elsevier; 2018. p. 155–96.

45. Pacheva IH, Ivanov IS. Migraine variants–occurrence in pediatric neurology practice. Clin Neurol Neurosurg 2013;115(9):1775–83.

46. Bosemani T, Burton VJ, Felling RJ, et al. Pediatric hemiplegic migraine: role of multiple MRI techniques in evaluation of reversible hypoperfusion. Cephalalgia 2014;34(4):311–5.

47. Fedak EM, Zumberge NA, Heyer GL. The diagnostic role for susceptibility-weighted MRI during sporadic hemiplegic migraine. Cephalalgia 2013;33(15):1258–63.

48. Altinok D, Agarwal A, Ascadi G, et al. Pediatric hemiplegic migraine: susceptibility weighted and MR perfusion imaging abnormality. Pediatr Radiol 2010;40(12):1958–61.

49. Lehman LL, Danehy AR, Trenor CC 3rd, et al. Transient focal neurologic symptoms correspond to regional cerebral hypoperfusion by MRI: a stroke mimic in children. AJNR Am J Neuroradiol 2017;38(11):2199–202.

50. Moharir M, Shroff M, Benseler SM. Childhood central nervous system vasculitis. Neuroimaging Clin N Am 2013;23(2):293–308.

51. Aviv RI, Benseler SM, Silverman ED, et al. MR imaging and angiography of primary CNS vasculitis of childhood. AJNR Am J Neuroradiol 2006;27(1):192–9.

52. Mandell DM, Mossa-Basha M, Qiao Y, et al. Intracranial vessel wall MRI: principles and expert consensus recommendations of the American Society of Neuroradiology. AJNR Am J Neuroradiol 2017;38(2):218–29.

53. Wasay M, Dai AI, Ansari M, et al. Cerebral venous sinus thrombosis in children: a multicenter cohort from the United States. J Child Neurol 2008;23(1):26–31.

54. Hedlund GL. Cerebral sinovenous thrombosis in pediatric practice. Pediatr Radiol 2013;43(2):173–88.

55. Bartynski WS. Posterior reversible encephalopathy syndrome, part 1: fundamental imaging and clinical features. AJNR Am J Neuroradiol 2008;29(6):1036–42.

56. Gupta V, Bhatia V, Khandelwal N, et al. Imaging findings in pediatric posterior reversible encephalopathy syndrome (PRES): 5 years of experience from a Tertiary Care Center in India. J Child Neurol 2016;31(9):1166–73.

57. Habetz K, Ramakrishnaiah R, Raina SK, et al. Posterior reversible encephalopathy syndrome: a comparative study of pediatric versus adult patients. Pediatr Neurol 2016;65:45–51.

58. Osborn AG. Acquired metabolic and systemic disorders. In: Osborn AG, Hedlund GL, Salzman KL, editors. Osborn's brain: imaging, pathology, and

anatomy. 2nd edition. Philadelphia: Elsevier; 2018. p. 1017–70.

59. Seol HJ, Wang KC, Kim SK, et al. Headache in pediatric moyamoya disease: review of 204 consecutive cases. J Neurosurg 2005;103(5 Suppl):439–42.

60. Zun Z, Hargreaves BA, Rosenberg J, et al. Improved multislice perfusion imaging with velocity-selective arterial spin labeling. J Magn Reson Imaging 2015; 41(5):1422–31.

61. Schwedt TJ, Guo Y, Rothner AD. "Benign" imaging abnormalities in children and adolescents with headache. Headache 2006;46(3):387–98.

62. Tubbs RS, McGirt MJ, Oakes WJ. Surgical experience in 130 pediatric patients with Chiari I malformations. J Neurosurg 2003;99(2):291–6.

63. Wu YW, Chin CT, Chan KM, et al. Pediatric Chiari I malformations: do clinical and radiologic features correlate? Neurology 1999;53(6):1271–6.

64. Fakhri A, Shah MN, Goyal MS. Advanced imaging of Chiari 1 malformations. Neurosurg Clin N Am 2015; 26(4):519–26.

65. Osborn AG. Nonneoplastic cysts. In: Osborn AG, Hedlund GL, Salzman KL, editors. Osborn's brain: imaging, pathology, and anatomy. 2nd edition. Philadelphia: Elsevier; 2018. p. 867–901.

66. Wu X, Li G, Zhao J, et al. Arachnoid cyst-associated chronic subdural hematoma: report of 14 cases and a systematic literature review. World Neurosurg 2018;109:e118–30.

67. Kraya T, Deschauer M, Joshi PR, et al. Prevalence of headache in patients with mitochondrial disease: a cross-sectional study. Headache 2018; 58(1):45–52.

68. Malhotra K, Liebeskind DS. Imaging of MELAS. Curr Pain Headache Rep 2016;20(9):54.

69. Rogers DL. A review of pediatric idiopathic intracranial hypertension. Pediatr Clin North Am 2014;61(3): 579–90.

70. Hartmann AJ, Soares BP, Bruce BB, et al. Imaging features of idiopathic intracranial hypertension in children. J Child Neurol 2017;32(1):120–6.

Headache and Brain Tumor

Shahram Hadidchi, MD[a], Wesley Surento, MS[a], Alexander Lerner, MD[a],
Chia-Shang Jason Liu, MD, PhD[a], Wende N. Gibbs, MD, MA[a], Paul E. Kim, MD[a],
Mark S. Shiroishi, MD, MS[b],*

KEYWORDS

- Pediatric and adult brain tumor • Primary headache • Secondary headache
- Pathophysiology of brain tumor headache • Brain tumor treatment

KEY POINTS

- The majority headache patients will not have a brain tumor. However, the presence of clinical "red flags" should further investigation with neuroimaging.
- Brain tumors are an uncommon cause of headaches in children and adults, however, many brain tumors do present with headache, typically accompanied by other neurological signs and symptoms.
- Recent guidelines from the American College of Radiology are an excellent resource regarding the appropriate the use of neuroimaging for headaches in children and adults.

INTRODUCTION

Headaches are exceedingly common. A highly-cited general population prevalence study by Rasmussen and colleagues[1] found that the lifetime prevalence of headache in any form in the general population was 93% for men and 99% for women, with the point prevalence being 11% for men and 22% for women. Most headaches are primary headache disorders comprised mainly of tension (69%–88%), migraine (6%–25%), and cluster headaches (0.006%–0.24%).[1,2] Most individuals seeking medical attention for headaches have no serious or life-threatening underlying pathologies,[3] but many are concerned about this possibility.[4] A large case-control study[5] suggested that isolated headache presenting in the primary care setting did not justify further investigation, because the risk of an underlying brain tumor was too small.

Likewise, the prevalence of asymptomatic brain tumors on neuroimaging studies is similarly low, estimated to be 0.7% (95% confidence interval [CI] 0.47%–0.98%) based on a meta-analysis of 16 studies (n = 19,559).[6]

The term atypical headache can be applied to those that are similar to primary headaches but have atypical features or clinical course. Although there are no definitive prevalence estimates of atypical headaches, one study found that major MR imaging abnormalities were found in 14.1% of atypical headache cases, while they were found in only 1.4% of tension-type and 0.6% of migraine headaches.[7] As opposed to primary headaches, the term secondary headaches refers to those with underlying pathologies such as intracranial tumor, infection, ruptured aneurysm, or giant cell arteritis. Secondary headaches are far less common than primary headaches.[8]

Admin Assistant: Kevin Pacheco. kevinpac@med.usc.edu.

M.S. Shiroishi was partially supported by NIH 1 L30 CA209248-01, Wright Foundation, American Cancer Society, Canon Medical Systems and the L. K. Whittier Foundation.

[a] Division of Neuroradiology, Department of Radiology, Keck School of Medicine, University of Southern California, 1520 San Pablo Street, Lower Level Imaging L1600, Los Angeles, CA 90033, USA; [b] Division of Neuroradiology, Department of Radiology, USC Imaging Genetics Center, Mark and Mary Stevens Neuroimaging and Informatics Institute, Keck School of Medicine of USC, University of Southern California, 1520 San Pablo Street, Lower Level Imaging L1600, Los Angeles, CA 90033, USA

* Corresponding author.

E-mail address: Mark.Shiroishi@med.usc.edu

This article describes the characteristics of headaches related to brain tumors in adults and children, provides neuroimaging recommendations in headache patients, and discusses the proposed pathophysiology and treatment of brain tumor-related headache.

HEADACHE IN ADULTS WITH BRAIN TUMORS

An underlying brain tumor is one of the most feared etiologies of headache, and, although brain tumors are an uncommon cause of headache,[9,10] many patients with brain tumors do complain of headaches.[10] The prevalence of headache in brain tumor patients ranges between 32.2% and 71% in unselected cases, and metastatic and primary brain tumors are equally likely to cause headaches.[11–16] Interestingly, there are anecdotal reports of patients with large intracranial tumors with increased intracranial pressure but no headache symptoms.[10] It is important to keep in mind that brain tumor-related headaches rarely present in isolation.[11,14,17] These headaches commonly present with other neurologic signs and symptoms like seizures, nausea/vomiting, personality changes, papilledema, blurred vision, and other focal neurologic deficits.[18,19] A change in the character of the headache, new symptoms, or progression are also concerning for an underlying brain tumor.[13]

The most recent International Classification of Headache Disroders-3[20] has defined "headache attributed to intracranial neoplasia" as one that occurs in a patient in whom an intracranial neoplasm has been diagnosed and in whom there is "evidence of causation demonstrated by one or more of the following: headache has developed in temporal relation to the intracranial neoplasia, or led to its discovery; headache has significantly worsened in parallel with worsening of the intracranial neoplasia; headache has significantly improved in temporal relation to successful treatment of the intracranial neoplasia; not better accounted for by another ICHD-3 diagnosis." The classic brain tumor headache has been described as severe, worse in the morning, and accompanied by nausea and vomiting.[12] An early clinical study of adult brain tumor headache was by Forsyth and Posner[12] in 1993 from Memorial Sloan-Kettering Cancer Center. They evaluated 111 consecutive brain tumor patients of whom 34% had primary brain tumors, and 66% had metastatic tumors. They found that 48% of primary and metastatic brain tumor patients presented with headaches and that the classic brain tumor headache was actually uncommon in their experience. Headaches were similar to tension-type in

77% of cases, migraine in 9% of cases, and other types in 14% of cases. However, unlike actual tension-type headaches, brain tumor headaches were worse with bending over in 32% of cases, while vomiting was seen 40% of the time. The headaches similar to tension-type headaches were described as dull ache, pressure, and like a sinus headache. Furthermore, larger tumors with contrast enhancement and midline shift were more likely to produce headaches, although the headache characteristics were nonspecific. The headaches were usually described as bilateral, but in those who had unilateral pain, the pain was always on the same side as the brain tumor. This finding was confirmed on a subsequent study from Thailand that found that this was highly predictive in both supra- and infratentorial tumors when there was no evidence of raised intracranial pressure.[15] In cases where intracranial pressure is elevated, tumor localization based on headache location becomes more difficult, likely because of widespread activation of pain receptors of the head.[10] Work from the early 1970s using electrical stimulation to the dura seemed to indicate that pain can be felt throughout the head and neck region.[21] This supports the general notion that determining tumor location based on headache distribution is imperfect, and with the availability of modern neuroimaging, this question can be easily answered.[10]

A 2007 study by Schankin and colleagues[14] of 85 patients with primary and metastatic tumors found that a pre-existing primary headache disorder could predispose to having a secondary brain tumor-related headache. The authors also suggested that an absence of raised intracranial pressure (such as could be seen after steroid treatment) could be responsible for the absence of classic brain tumor findings. They also suggested that glioblastoma patients had more dull headaches, while those with meningioma had pulsating headaches. An important prospective study by Valentinis and colleagues[16] in 2010 in 206 patients found that brain tumor headache prevalence was 47.6% and that the headache was nonspecific in character and that its prevalence differed according to tumor location, volume, and the patient's prior headache history. Like other studies,[13,15] they also found that infratentorial tumors were more commonly associated with headaches, likely because of the small size of the posterior fossa and CSF flow obstruction.[19]

Brain metastases are by far the most common brain tumors in adults, and in adults with a cancer history, a new or changed headache without other neurologic signs or symptoms can be associated with brain metastases in up to

54% of patients.[18,22] In children with a cancer history and new headache, the risk of intracranial metastatic diseases has been reported to be 12%.[23]

SELECTED BRAIN TUMOR HEADACHE SYNDROMES

Although a tumor's type, location, and size may not be predictably related to headache, there are some characteristic headache syndromes that appear to be associated with tumor location.[24,25]

Metastatic tumors to the skull base can elicit distinct clinical syndromes related to their location:[19,26]

- Orbital: dull unilateral supraorbital headache, diplopia, ptosis, V1 distribution trigeminal sensory loss
- Parasellar: unilateral frontal headache, V1 distribution sensory loss, diplopia, and ocular paresis
- Occipital condyle: severe unilateral occipital pain worsened with neck flexion and unilateral tongue paralysis
- Jugular foramen: unilateral retroauricular pain, IX to XI cranial nerve paralysis, hoarseness, and dysphagia
- Gasserian ganglion syndrome: trigeminal neural-like pain in forehead, cheek or jaw, and V2 or V3 distribution sensory loss

Trigeminal autonomic cephalgias (TACs) are primary headache syndromes comprised of severe short-lasting headaches along with paroxysmal facial autonomic symptoms.[27] Pituitary tumors have an unusual association with TACs, and so those presenting with this uncommon headache disorder should be considered for further work-up.[25] In an another context related to the pituitary gland, pituitary apoplexy is a well-known severe consequence of infarction/hemorrhage of a pituitary tumor. This is classically associated with acute severe headache, sometimes characterized as thunderclap, along with focal neurologic deficits including visual loss and potentially death from pituitary insufficiency.[28–33] Urgent surgery and glucocorticoid therapy are important to avoid serious complications; however, those with asymptomatic apoplexy may have good outcomes with tumor-specific and steroid treatments.[33,34]

Several cystic intracranial masses merit discussion. Colloid cysts classically produce severe acute headaches relieved by positional changes,[35] although more recent studies suggest that they more commonly cause intermittent diffuse headaches, often unrelated to position.[36] Acute obstruction at the foramen of Monro can be associated with severe consequences including death due to hydrocephalus.[28] Other cystic intracranial lesions such as anteroinferior middle cranial fossa arachnoid cysts may produce a nummular headache (left temporal headache location).[37] Supra- and intrasellar arachnoid cysts may produce unilateral cluster headache,[38] and large right frontal arachnoid cysts without hydrocephalus can produce occipital orgasmic headache.[39] When pineal cysts grow large enough to produce hydrocephalus, they may produce headache; however, it is theorized that those that are too small to result in hydrocephalus may still produce headache. After pinealectomy, these patients may still complain of unilateral headache with or without autonomic features and visual symptoms.[40] Melatonin is thought to have anti-inflammatory properties, and it is thought that tumors that infiltrate the pineal gland like germinoma can result in a decrease in melatonin, while other tumors like pinealoblastoma and pinealocytoma may actually increase levels of melatonin.[41] Other intracranial masses such as dermoid/epidermoid tumors and craniopharyngiomas may produce headache secondary to a chemical meningitis secondary to a rupture of their contents into the CSF.[37–39]

NEUROIMAGING RECOMMENDATIONS IN ADULTS WITH HEADACHE

Evaluation of the adult headache patient begins with a thorough history and physical examination. A useful resource regarding the use of neuroimaging in a headache patient is the American College of Radiology (ACR) Appropriateness Criteria Headache,[42] which provides evidence-based guidelines for physicians. The ACR recommends that most patients who present with non-traumatic, uncomplicated primary headache do not need neuroimaging. However, those who present with concerning red flags based on history or physical examination should be considered for neuroimaging to exclude an underlying secondary cause like a brain tumor. It is important for the physician to consider other serious intracranial disorders that could result in headache.[25] These are outlined in **Box 1**.

For patients with chronic headache, the ACR recommends that new headache features and/or focal neurologic signs/symptoms could suggest an underlying brain tumor, aneurysm, or vascular malformation, and in these cases contrast-enhanced brain MR imaging should be

---

Box 1

Differential diagnoses to consider other than brain tumor in a headache patient

Other space-occupying processes (eg, hematoma or abscess)

Subarachnoid hemorrhage

Infection including encephalitis, meningitis

Traumatic head injury

Serious otolaryngologic and ophthalmologic causes of headache

Stroke (intracerebral hemorrhage, infarction, cerebral venous thrombosis)

Temporal arteritis

Box 2

Clinical red flags warranting further evaluation with neuroimaging

Headaches that occur immediately after waking at night or awaken patient repeatedly from sleep

Headache with new neurologic signs

Headache that is progressive

Acute headache or persistent headache without associated family history of migraine

Acute new, usually severe, headache or headache that has changed from prior headaches

Acute headache following strenuous exercise

Headache associated with fever or other systemic symptoms

Headache with meningismus

Headache with Valsalva maneuver (by bending down, coughing, sneezing, or straining)

New headache in an adult, especially over 50 years of age

New headache in the elderly or children

Headaches not characteristic of primary headaches

Headaches associated with vomiting/nausea without migraine

Blurred vision, diplopia, papilledema

New or changed headache in a cancer patient

Chronic headaches occurring with substantial disorientation, confusion, or emesis

Unilateral headache associated with contralateral neurologic symptoms

Focal neurologic symptoms other than sensory or visual aura

---

considered.[42] Other situations where neuroimaging may be indicated is with new headache in immunosuppressed or cancer patients because of the increased risk of infection or brain tumor. Various publications have proposed clinical red flags that should raise the suspicion of a serious underlying cause including brain tumor.[10,25,43] These are summarized in **Box 2**.

HEADACHE IN CHILDREN WITH BRAIN TUMORS

Brain tumors are the most common solid tumors of childhood and the leading cause of cancer death from ages 0 to 14 years in the United States.[44,45] The clinical presentation of pediatric brain tumors has been less studied than in adults.[46] Children with brain tumors frequently present with headaches, although their presentation may be less clear or complete relative to adults.[47] Brain tumor headaches in children, as in adults, are often associated with other neurologic signs and symptoms[14] (**Box 1**). Early diagnosis is critical to improving outcomes, but pediatric brain tumors are often initially misdiagnosed as more common pediatric disorders like migraine, gastroenteritis, or psychological/behavioral conditions.[48] Similarly, given the lack of pathognomonic clinical features of brain tumors in children, there has been no significant change in the prediagnostic interval in the last several decades despite widespread availability of computed tomography (CT) and MR imaging.

A large series[46] of 200 children with brain tumors found that the most common initial presenting symptoms were headache (41%), vomiting (12%), unsteadiness (11%), visual difficulties (10%), educational/behavioral problems (10%) and seizures (9%). The most common symptoms occurring at any time were headache (56%), vomiting (51%), and educational or behavioral problems (44%). Eighty-eight percent of subjects had neurologic signs at diagnosis including papilledema (38%), cranial nerve abnormalities (49%), cerebellar signs (48%), long tract signs (27%), somatosensory abnormalities (11%), and reduced level of consciousness (12%). More than 1 sign or symptom was present at the time of diagnosis except for seizures. Other older large series also found that children with brain tumors typically have other neurologic signs and symptoms in addition to headache.[49,50] A recent review has summarized common physical examination findings in pediatric brain tumor patients (**Box 3**).[48]

Despite the fact that brain tumors are the most common solid tumors of childhood, only rarely

---

Box 3

Common physical examination findings in children with brain tumors

Cranial Nerves

  Nystagmus

  Facial palsy

  Double vision

  Reduced hearing

  Abnormal eye movement

  Difficulty swallowing

  Head tilt

  Deviation of tongue

Others

  Paresis

  Hyper/o reflexia

  Increased/decreased muscle tone

  Positive Romberg sign

  Dysmetria

  Heel-knee-shin ataxia

  Papilledema

  Clonus

---

will a child with a headache actually have a brain tumor. In a series of 105 children younger than 6 years with chronic and recurrent headaches, Raieli and colleagues[51] found only 3 (2.85%) cases with brain tumors. Another series of 104 children younger than 7 years with headache, the most common reason was migraine, and no brain tumor was found in their patients.[52] In a large series of 815 children younger than 18 years with chronic headache, Abu-Arafeh and Macleod[53] reported only 2 patients with brain tumors. A relatively recent series of 51 children with craniopharyngioma found that 78% of their subjects reported headache and that this was associated with hydrocephalus, distortion of circle of Willis, and large tumor volume.[54] Both distortion of the circle of Willis and large tumor volume were also associated with greater frequency and severity of headaches.

NEUROIMAGING RECOMMENDATIONS IN CHILDREN WITH HEADACHE

Although an actual underlying brain tumor is rare in a child, headaches can understandably result in enough concern from a clinician or parent to warrant neuroimaging.[55,56] As with adults, a thorough history and physical examination are vital in order to elicit whether red flags (see **Box 1**) are present. As with adults, the ACR recently published its evidenced-based guidelines regarding neuroimaging of children with headaches.[56]

The most common types of headache in children are primary headaches such as migraine or tension headaches. However, pediatric migraine headaches may differ from those in adults (eg, they may be of shorter duration in children).[57,58] The neuroimaging yield of clinically significant findings in pediatric patients with primary headaches is low.[55,59–63] Younger children are more likely to have secondary headaches, and while most have a benign cause, chronic progressive headaches, along with abnormal physical examination findings, could indicate an underlying brain tumor.[51,64] Imaging should be considered in those with nonspecific symptoms and normal physical examination results if there is not typical resolution of symptoms.[48] Urgent imaging should be particularly considered in those with paresis and unsteadiness. A summary of general guidelines for neuroimaging of headache that incorporates the ACR guidelines,[42,56] the American Academy of Neurology and Child Neurology Society,[65] and systematic review of neuroimaging in childhood headache[55] are summarized in **Box 4**.

Box 4

Recommendations for neuroimaging in children with headache

- Neuroimaging is usually not appropriate for the initial imaging of primary headache in children.

- In cases of secondary headache, noncontrast-enhanced brain MR imaging is usually appropriate, and a contrast-enhanced examination should be obtained if the noncontrast examination is abnormal.

- There are tradeoffs regarding the use of CT versus MR imaging in the neuroimaging of children. Children are exposed ionizing radiation with CT, while sedation or general anesthesia is sometimes needed for MR imaging examinations in children younger than 6 years. Given this, careful consideration is needed, and neuroimaging should be conducted in only those children with suspicious history and physical examination findings that point to serious intracranial pathology.

- If brain MR imaging reveals a brain tumor in a child, a contrast-enhanced MR imaging of the entire spine to exclude drop metastasis should be considered, especially for tumors of the posterior fossa.

PATHOPHYSIOLOGY OF HEADACHE IN BRAIN TUMORS

The brain parenchyma itself is insensitive to pain because it lacks pain receptors. However, the tissues covering the cranium, including the periosteum of the skull, muscles, vessels, skin/subcutaneous tissues; eye, ear paranasal sinuses, and nasal cavity; dural venous sinuses; pia arachnoid and dura mater; trigeminal, glossopharyngeal, vagus, and first 3 cervical nerves are sensitive to mechanical stimulation.[17] It is generally thought that displacement and traction of these sensitive intracranial structures underlie brain tumor-related headaches. Raised intracranial pressure results in traction due to brain tumor edema, tumor expansion, and hemorrhage.[66] The clinicoradiologic correlates of increased intracranial pressure including midline shift, papilledema, and peritumoral edema are typically associated with poorly localized diffuse headaches.[12,13] However, this relationship is imperfectly understood, and further work, including that focusing on serologic, cerebral, and CSF factors is needed to better define the pathophysiology.[10]

Brain tumor headaches can sometimes be intense but temporary because of transitory ventricular system obstruction from the tumor induced by exertion, postural change, Valsalva maneuver, and coughing.[10] An abnormal cerebrovascular autoregulatory response to vasodilation related to raised intracranial pressure and/or space-occupying event is another postulated mechanism of acute brain tumor headaches.[10]

The growth rate of brain tumors can also influence the characteristics of headaches.[13,19,66] Because slow-growing tumors can allow adaptation to mass effect, they can produce transitory headaches later in the disease process. On the other hand, fast-growing tumors do not allow adaptation and so can result in intense, sharp pain.

Brain tumor location may also impact whether a headache is produced. Brain tumors that are midline, intraventricular, and posterior fossa in location are generally known to result in headaches due to CSF flow obstruction.[11,13,15,66] Although cranial nerves and cervical nerve roots are sensitive to pain, nerve compression itself is rarely thought to result in brain tumor headache.[11] However, when cervical nerve compression appears to be associated with brain tumor headache, it can be seen along with the presence of myofascial trigger points and muscle tenderness, likely triggered by external pressure or neck movements.[10]

In certain situations, little or no direct mass effect on pain-sensitive structures from tumors might result in brain tumor headaches. This is thought to be due to endocrinological etiologies, such as with pituitary tumors where somatostatin and dopamine may have a potential proprioceptive role in the development of headache.[67,68] Other publications posit that pituitary tumors cause headaches because of a cavernous sinus invasion and dural stretching.[69] Other possible causes of brain tumor headaches include substances produced by brain tumors such as tachykinin (substance P), calcitonin gene-related peptide, nitric oxide synthase, tumor necrosis factor alpha, and vasoactive intestinal peptide.[24]

Finally, the treatment of brain tumors itself can result in headache, and these factors are summarized in **Box 5**.[70] Several surgical series have reported a high incidence of postcraniotomy headache, both immediately and remote,[71–75] especially in the case of retrosigmoid craniotomy.[76] Radiation therapy of the brain can result in immediate or remote headache and can be associated with worsening of neurologic function.[77] Cerebral radiation necrosis can occur months to years after initial treatment and can be associated with focal neurologic deficits and headache.[25] In high-grade glioma patients treated with temozolomide chemoradiation, increased edema and contrast-enhancement immediately after treatment can worsen symptoms and result in headaches.[78] Temozolomide itself has also been associated with headache in glioblastoma patients.[79] Other agents used in the treatment of brain tumors such as corticosteroids and antinausea agents like ondansetron[80] and bevacizumab[81] are also known to result in headaches.

TREATMENT OF BRAIN TUMOR HEADACHES

For brain tumor patients with headache, treatment of the underlying neoplasm improves the headache in most cases.[13,16,82,83] Because patients

---

Box 5
Brain tumor treatment factors associated with headache

Craniotomy

Radiation therapy – both acute and remote, including radiation necrosis

Chemotherapy agents (eg, temozolomide)

Corticosteroids

Bevacizumab

Antinausea agents (eg, ondansetron)

with a history of a primary headache disorder more commonly suffer from brain tumor-related headaches,[12,16] if a headache appears to be primary, rather than secondary in a brain tumor patient, conventional therapy for the primary headache is warranted.[25] Medical therapy with analgesics and opiates is commonly used,[24,25] and in cases with highly aggressive brain malignancies, adequate pain control is central to quality of life. Control of hydrocephalus with intracranial pressure monitoring and ventricular shunting and management of cerebral edema are key initial treatment strategies before chemotherapy, radiotherapy, or surgical therapy.[24] Corticosteroid treatment for cerebral edema can result in substantial transient improvement of headache. In patients with cerebral metastases, whole-brain radiation may improve headache symptoms and decrease corticosteroid usage.[84,85] Surgical resection or stereotactic radiosurgery for those with a few metastases can also result in control of headache.[86–88]

SUMMARY

Most headache patients will not have life-threatening illnesses like a brain tumor. However, the clinician must perform a careful history and physical examination for the presence of red flags that would warrant neuroimaging. Brain tumors are an uncommon cause of headaches in children and adults; however, many brain tumors do present with headache, typically accompanied by other neurologic signs and symptoms. Early diagnosis of pediatric brain tumors remains especially difficult, because they can be initially misdiagnosed as more common benign disorders. Generally, the treatment of the underlying brain tumor improves the headache; however, these therapies may also induce headaches. The recent evidence-based guidelines from the ACR[42,56] serve as an excellent resource for clinicians regarding the use neuroimaging for headaches in children and adults.

REFERENCES

1. Rasmussen BK, Jensen R, Schroll M, et al. Epidemiology of headache in a general population–a prevalence study. J Clin Epidemiol 1991;44(11):1147–57.
2. Dousset V, Henry P, Michel P. Epidemiology of headache. Rev Neurol (Paris) 2000;156(Suppl 4):4S24–9 [in French].
3. Kernick D, Stapley S, Goadsby PJ, et al. What happens to new-onset headache presented to primary care? A case-cohort study using electronic primary care records. Cephalalgia 2008;28(11):1188–95.
4. Kurth T, Buring JE, Rist PM. Headache, migraine and risk of brain tumors in women: prospective cohort study. J Headache Pain 2015;16:501.
5. Hamilton W, Kernick D. Clinical features of primary brain tumours: a case-control study using electronic primary care records. Br J Gen Pract 2007;57(542):695–9.
6. Morris Z, Whiteley WN, Longstreth WT Jr, et al. Incidental findings on brain magnetic resonance imaging: systematic review and meta-analysis. BMJ 2009;339:b3016.
7. Wang HZ, Simonson TM, Greco WR, et al. Brain MR imaging in the evaluation of chronic headache in patients without other neurologic symptoms. Acad Radiol 2001;8(5):405–8.
8. Frishberg BM, Rosenberg JH, Matchar DB, et al. Evidence-based guidelines in the primary care setting: neuroimaging in patients with nonacute headache 2000. Available at: tools.aan.com/professionals/practice/pdfs/gl0088.pdf.
9. Taylor LP. Mechanism of brain tumor headache. Headache 2014;54(4):772–5.
10. Goffaux P, Fortin D. Brain tumor headaches: from bedside to bench. Neurosurgery 2010;67(2):459–66.
11. Vazquez-Barquero A, Ibanez FJ, Herrera S, et al. Isolated headache as the presenting clinical manifestation of intracranial tumors: a prospective study. Cephalalgia 1994;14(4):270–2.
12. Forsyth PA, Posner JB. Headaches in patients with brain tumors: a study of 111 patients. Neurology 1993;43(9):1678–83.
13. Pfund Z, Szapary L, Jaszberenyi O, et al. Headache in intracranial tumors. Cephalalgia 1999;19(9):787–90 [discussion: 765].
14. Schankin CJ, Ferrari U, Reinisch VM, et al. Characteristics of brain tumour-associated headache. Cephalalgia 2007;27(8):904–11.
15. Suwanwela N, Phanthumchinda K, Kaoropthum S. Headache in brain tumor: a cross-sectional study. Headache 1994;34(7):435–8.
16. Valentinis L, Tuniz F, Valent F, et al. Headache attributed to intracranial tumours: a prospective cohort study. Cephalalgia 2010;30(4):389–98.
17. Boiardi A, Salmaggi A, Eoli M, et al. Headache in brain tumours: a symptom to reappraise critically. Neurol Sci 2004;25(Suppl 3):S143–7.
18. Christiaans MH, Kelder JC, Arnoldus EP, et al. Prediction of intracranial metastases in cancer patients with headache. Cancer 2002;94(7):2063–8.
19. Loghin M, Levin VA. Headache related to brain tumors. Curr Treat Options Neurol 2006;8(1):21–32.
20. Society TIH. The International classification of headache disorders. 3rd edition 2018. Available at: https://www.ichd-3.org/.

21. Wirth FP Jr, Van Buren JM. Referral of pain from dural stimulation in man. J Neurosurg 1971;34(5): 630–42.

22. Argyriou AA, Chroni E, Polychronopoulos P, et al. Headache characteristics and brain metastases prediction in cancer patients. Eur J Cancer Care (Engl) 2006;15(1):90–5.

23. Antunes NL. The spectrum of neurologic disease in children with systemic cancer. Pediatr Neurol 2001; 25(3):227–35.

24. Kahn K, Finkel A. It is a tumor – current review of headache and brain tumor. Curr Pain Headache Rep 2014;18(6):421.

25. Kirby S, Purdy RA. Headaches and brain tumors. Neurol Clin 2014;32(2):423–32.

26. Greenberg HS, Deck MD, Vikram B, et al. Metastasis to the base of the skull: clinical findings in 43 patients. Neurology 1981;31(5):530–7.

27. Favier I, van Vliet JA, Roon KI, et al. Trigeminal autonomic cephalgias due to structural lesions: a review of 31 cases. Arch Neurol 2007;64(1):25–31.

28. de Witt Hamer PC, Verstegen MJ, De Haan RJ, et al. High risk of acute deterioration in patients harboring symptomatic colloid cysts of the third ventricle. J Neurosurg 2002;96(6):1041–5.

29. Satoh H, Uozumi T, Arita K, et al. Spontaneous rupture of craniopharyngioma cysts. A report of five cases and review of the literature. Surg Neurol 1993;40(5):414–9.

30. Gormley WB, Tomecek FJ, Qureshi N, et al. Craniocerebral epidermoid and dermoid tumours: a review of 32 cases. Acta Neurochir (Wien) 1994;128(1–4):115–21.

31. Stendel R, Pietila TA, Lehmann K, et al. Ruptured intracranial dermoid cysts. Surg Neurol 2002;57(6): 391–8 [discussion: 398].

32. Levy MJ, Jager HR, Powell M, et al. Pituitary volume and headache: size is not everything. Arch Neurol 2004;61(5):721–5.

33. Nawar RN, AbdelMannan D, Selman WR, et al. Pituitary tumor apoplexy: a review. J Intensive Care Med 2008;23(2):75–90.

34. Chen L, White WL, Spetzler RF, et al. A prospective study of nonfunctioning pituitary adenomas: presentation, management, and clinical outcome. J Neurooncol 2011;102(1):129–38.

35. Harris W. Paroxysmal and postural headaches from intraventricular cysts and tumors. Lancet 1944;2: 654–5.

36. Desai KI, Nadkarni TD, Muzumdar DP, et al. Surgical management of colloid cyst of the third ventricle–a study of 105 cases. Surg Neurol 2002;57(5): 295–302 [discussion: 302–4].

37. Guillem A, Barriga FJ, Gimenez-Roldan S. Nummular headache associated to arachnoid cysts. J Headache Pain 2009;10(3):215–7.

38. Edvardsson B, Persson S. Cluster headache and arachnoid cyst. Springerplus 2013;2(1):4.

39. Kang SY, Choi JC, Kang JH, et al. Huge supratentorial arachnoid cyst presenting as an orgasmic headache. Neurol Sci 2012;33(3):639–41.

40. Chazot G, Claustrat B, Broussolle E, et al. Headache and depression: recurrent symptoms in adult pinealectomized patients. In: Nappi G, Al E, editors. Headache and depression: serotonin pathways as a common clue. New York: Raven Press; 1991. p. 299–303.

41. Claustrat B, Brun J, Chazot G. The basic physiology and pathophysiology of melatonin. Sleep Med Rev 2005;9(1):11–24.

42. Douglas AC, Wippold FJ 2nd, Broderick DF, et al. ACR appropriateness criteria headache. J Am Coll Radiol 2014;11(7):657–67.

43. Purdy RA. Clinical evaluation of a patient presenting with headache. Med Clin North Am 2001;85(4): 847–63, v.

44. Linabery AM, Ross JA. Trends in childhood cancer incidence in the U.S. (1992-2004). Cancer 2008; 112(2):416–32.

45. Ostrom QT, de Blank PM, Kruchko C, et al. Alex's Lemonade Stand Foundation infant and childhood primary brain and central nervous system tumors diagnosed in the United States in 2007-2011. Neuro Oncol 2015;16(Suppl 10):x1–36.

46. Wilne SH, Ferris RC, Nathwani A, et al. The presenting features of brain tumours: a review of 200 cases. Arch Dis Child 2006;91(6):502–6.

47. Punt J. Clinical syndromes. In: Walker D, Perilongo G, Punt J, editors. Brain and spinal tumours of childhood. London: Arnold; 2004. p. 99–106.

48. Goldman RD, Cheng S, Cochrane DD. Improving diagnosis of pediatric central nervous system tumours: aiming for early detection. CMAJ 2017; 189(12):E459–63.

49. The epidemiology of headache among children with brain tumor. Headache in children with brain tumors. The Childhood Brain Tumor Consortium. J Neurooncol 1991;10(1):31–46.

50. Medina LS, Pinter JD, Zurakowski D, et al. Children with headache: clinical predictors of surgical space-occupying lesions and the role of neuroimaging. Radiology 1997;202(3):819–24.

51. Raieli V, Eliseo M, Pandolfi E, et al. Recurrent and chronic headaches in children below 6 years of age. J Headache Pain 2005;6(3):135–42.

52. Chu M, Shinnar S. Headaches in children younger than 7 years of age. Arch Neurol 1992; 49(1):79–82.

53. Abu-Arafeh I, Macleod S. Serious neurological disorders in children with chronic headache. Arch Dis Child 2005;90(9):937–40.

54. Khan RB, Merchant TE, Boop FA, et al. Headaches in children with craniopharyngioma. J Child Neurol 2013;28(12):1622–5.

55. Alexiou GA, Argyropoulou MI. Neuroimaging in childhood headache: a systematic review. Pediatr Radiol 2013;43(7):777–84.

56. Expert Panel on Pediatric I, Hayes LL, Palasis S, et al. ACR appropriateness criteria((R)) headache-child. J Am Coll Radiol 2018;15(5S):S78–90.

57. Lateef TM, Grewal M, McClintock W, et al. Headache in young children in the emergency department: use of computed tomography. Pediatrics 2009;124(1):e12–7.

58. Arruda MA, Guidetti V, Galli F, et al. Primary headaches in childhood–a population-based study. Cephalalgia 2010;30(9):1056–64.

59. Schwedt TJ, Guo Y, Rothner AD. "Benign" imaging abnormalities in children and adolescents with headache. Headache 2006;46(3):387–98.

60. Sempere AP, Porta-Etessam J, Medrano V, et al. Neuroimaging in the evaluation of patients with non-acute headache. Cephalalgia 2005;25(1):30–5.

61. DeVries A, Young PC, Wall E, et al. CT scan utilization patterns in pediatric patients with recurrent headache. Pediatrics 2013;132(1):e1–8.

62. Martens D, Oster I, Gottschlling S, et al. Cerebral MRI and EEG studies in the initial management of pediatric headaches. Swiss Med Wkly 2012;142:w13625.

63. Yilmaz U, Celegen M, Yilmaz TS, et al. Childhood headaches and brain magnetic resonance imaging findings. Eur J Paediatr Neurol 2014;18(2):163–70.

64. Nallasamy K, Singhi SC, Singhi P. Approach to headache in emergency department. Indian J Pediatr 2012;79(3):376–80.

65. Lewis DW, Ashwal S, Dahl G, et al. Practice parameter: evaluation of children and adolescents with recurrent headaches: report of the Quality Standards Subcommittee of the American Academy of Neurology and the Practice Committee of the Child Neurology Society. Neurology 2002;59(4):490–8.

66. Kunkle EC, Ray BS, Wolff HG. Studies on headache: the mechanisms and significance of the headache associated with brain tumor. Bull N Y Acad Med 1942;18(6):400–22.

67. Williams G, Ball JA, Lawson RA, et al. Analgesic effect of somatostatin analogue (octreotide) in headache associated with pituitary tumours. Br Med J (Clin Res Ed) 1987;295(6592):247–8.

68. Levy MJ, Matharu MS, Goadsby PJ. Prolactinomas, dopamine agonists and headache: two case reports. Eur J Neurol 2003;10(2):169–73.

69. Levy MJ. The association of pituitary tumors and headache. Curr Neurol Neurosci Rep 2011;11(2):164–70.

70. Obermann M, Holle D, Naegel S, et al. Headache attributable to nonvascular intracranial disorders. Curr Pain Headache Rep 2011;15(4):314–23.

71. Rocha-Filho PA. Post-craniotomy headache: a clinical view with a focus on the persistent form. Headache 2015;55(5):733–8.

72. de Oliveira Ribeiro Mdo C, Pereira CU, Sallum AM, et al. Immediate post-craniotomy headache. Cephalalgia 2013;33(11):897–905.

73. Rocha-Filho PA, Fujarra FJ, Gherpelli JL, et al. The long-term effect of craniotomy on temporalis muscle function. Oral Surg Oral Med Oral Pathol Oral Radiol Endod 2007;104(5):e17–21.

74. Ryzenman JM, Pensak ML, Tew JM Jr. Headache: a quality of life analysis in a cohort of 1,657 patients undergoing acoustic neuroma surgery, results from the acoustic neuroma association. Laryngoscope 2005;115(4):703–11.

75. Rimaaja T, Haanpaa M, Blomstedt G, et al. Headaches after acoustic neuroma surgery. Cephalalgia 2007;27(10):1128–35.

76. Ansari SF, Terry C, Cohen-Gadol AA. Surgery for vestibular schwannomas: a systematic review of complications by approach. Neurosurg Focus 2012;33(3):E14.

77. Schultheiss TE, Kun LE, Ang KK, et al. Radiation response of the central nervous system. Int J Radiat Oncol Biol Phys 1995;31(5):1093–112.

78. Brandsma D, Stalpers L, Taal W, et al. Clinical features, mechanisms, and management of pseudoprogression in malignant gliomas. Lancet Oncol 2008;9(5):453–61.

79. Yung WK, Albright RE, Olson J, et al. A phase II study of temozolomide vs. procarbazine in patients with glioblastoma multiforme at first relapse. Br J Cancer 2000;83(5):588–93.

80. Kalaycio M, Mendez Z, Pohlman B, et al. Continuous-infusion granisetron compared to ondansetron for the prevention of nausea and vomiting after high-dose chemotherapy. J Cancer Res Clin Oncol 1998;124(5):265–9.

81. Lou E, Turner S, Sumrall A, et al. Bevacizumab-induced reversible posterior leukoencephalopathy syndrome and successful retreatment in a patient with glioblastoma. J Clin Oncol 2011;29(28):e739–42.

82. Schmidinger M, Linzmayer L, Becherer A, et al. Psychometric- and quality-of-life assessment in long-term glioblastoma survivors. J Neurooncol 2003;63(1):55–61.

83. Pace A, Di Lorenzo C, Guariglia L, et al. End of life issues in brain tumor patients. J Neurooncol 2009;91(1):39–43.

84. Steinmann D, Paelecke-Habermann Y, Geinitz H, et al. Prospective evaluation of quality of life effects in patients undergoing palliative radiotherapy for brain metastases. BMC Cancer 2012;12:283.

85. Wong J, Hird A, Zhang L, et al. Symptoms and quality of life in cancer patients with brain metastases

following palliative radiotherapy. Int J Radiat Oncol Biol Phys 2009;75(4):1125–31.

86. Patchell RA, Tibbs PA, Walsh JW, et al. A randomized trial of surgery in the treatment of single metastases to the brain. N Engl J Med 1990; 322(8):494–500.

87. Kondziolka D, Patel A, Lunsford LD, et al. Stereotactic radiosurgery plus whole brain radiotherapy versus radiotherapy alone for patients with multiple brain metastases. Int J Radiat Oncol Biol Phys 1999;45(2):427–34.

88. Sanghavi SN, Miranpuri SS, Chappell R, et al. Radiosurgery for patients with brain metastases: a multi-institutional analysis, stratified by the RTOG recursive partitioning analysis method. Int J Radiat Oncol Biol Phys 2001;51(2):426–34.

Advanced Imaging in the Evaluation of Migraine Headaches

Benjamin M. Ellingson, PhD[a,b,c,d,e,f,*],
Chelsea Hesterman, MD[g], Mollie Johnston, MD[g],
Nicholas R. Dudeck, BS[a,b], Andrew C. Charles, MD[g],
Juan Pablo Villablanca, MD[b]

KEYWORDS

• Advanced neuroimaging • Migraine • Aura • Pain processing network • Pain matrix

KEY POINTS

• Clinical use of advanced imaging in headaches is not standardized; no single diagnostic imaging technique is able to define and/or differentiate idiopathic headache syndromes.
• In migraine with aura, cortical thinning, microstructural changes, spatiotemporal fluctuations in blood flow, adaptations in brain function, and alterations in both metabolism and biochemistry have been observed in pain processing areas of the brain (thalamus, insula, amygdala, brainstem, hippocampus, prefrontal cortex, anterior cingulate cortex, cerebellum, supplemental motor area, primary and secondary somatosensory areas, and the posterior parietal cortex).
• A characteristic decrease in blood flow has been observed during aura, whereas a significant increase in blood flow has been observed in subsequent stages of migraine attacks.
• Imaging changes in migraine patients who do not experience aura are subtler and more complex, with studies varying widely in the literature.

INTRODUCTION

Headache is a common symptom with a wide variety of potential causes. More than 70% of the US population are estimated to experience headaches,[1,2] with most headaches being caused by benign primary headache disorders and not significant pathologic conditions.[1,3] Migraine is a severe, disabling brain condition that ranks as sixth most disabling disorder globally according to the World Health Organization.[4,5] Migraine is the

[a] UCLA Center for Computer Vision and Imaging Biomarkers, David Geffen School of Medicine, University of California Los Angeles, 924 Westwood Boulevard, Suite 615, Los Angeles, CA 90024, USA; [b] Department of Radiological Sciences, David Geffen School of Medicine, University of California Los Angeles, 924 Westwood Boulevard, Suite 615, Los Angeles, CA 90024, USA; [c] Department of Psychiatry and Biobehavioral Sciences, David Geffen School of Medicine, University of California Los Angeles, 760 Westwood Plaza, Los Angeles, CA 90095, USA; [d] UCLA Brain Research Institute (BRI), David Geffen School of Medicine, University of California Los Angeles, 695 Charles E Young Dr S, Los Angeles, CA 90095, USA; [e] UCLA Brain Tumor Imaging Laboratory (BTIL), Department of Radiological Sciences, David Geffen School of Medicine, University of California, Los Angeles, 924 Westwood Boulevard, Suite 615, Los Angeles, CA 90024, USA; [f] UCLA Brain Tumor Imaging Laboratory (BTIL), Department of Psychiatry, David Geffen School of Medicine, University of California, Los Angeles, 924 Westwood Boulevard, Suite 615, Los Angeles, CA 90024, USA; [g] Department of Neurology, David Geffen School of Medicine, University of California, Los Angeles, 710 Westwood Plaza, Los Angeles, CA 90095-1769, USA
* Corresponding author. UCLA Brain Tumor Imaging Laboratory (BTIL), Department of Psychiatry, David Geffen School of Medicine, University of California, Los Angeles, 924 Westwood Boulevard, Suite 615, Los Angeles, CA 90024.
E-mail address: bellingson@mednet.ucla.edu

Neuroimag Clin N Am 29 (2019) 301–324
https://doi.org/10.1016/j.nic.2019.01.009

most frequent neurologic disorder in adults, affecting up to 12% of the general population.[6] The annual costs of migraine, including lost productivity, are more than $19.6 billion in the United States[7] and €27 billion in Europe,[8] making it a significant public health issue.

The current pathophysiologic concepts of headache formation, including migraine, implicate vascular changes, including changes in vessel diameter and cerebral blood flow (CBF), as part of the migraine phenomenon[9]; however, to date no single diagnostic tool is able to define, ensure, or differentiate the various headache syndromes. Clinical use of neuroimaging in diagnosing headache varies widely, and the overall yield of neuroimaging studies to identify significant abnormalities in patients presenting with headache has been reported to be less than 8%.[2,3,10–14] Recommendations regarding when to perform imaging for headache have been published by the US Headache Consortium, American Academy of Neurology,[15] American College of Emergency Physicians,[16] and the American College of Radiology based on the current level of scientific and clinical evidence.[1,17] Consistent with most of these suggestions, the European Federation of Neurological Societies Task Force does not recommend routine use of neuroimaging in adult and pediatric patients with migraine with no recent change in attack pattern, seizures, or other focal neurologic symptoms,[18] highlighting the often contradictory and nonspecific findings in the literature. Despite these recommendations, MR imaging and PET imaging appear to have significant potential for exploring the pathophysiology of headaches and potentially determine the effects of therapeutic interventions.[18]

PAIN CIRCUITS IN MIGRAINE

During acute pain resulting from migraine or other pain conditions, focal increases in CBF have been found bilaterally within the anterior insula, contralateral thalamus, ipsilateral anterior cingulate cortex (ACC), and the cerebellum.[19] Activation of ACC has been reported in PET studies on sensation of somatic or visceral pain as well as emotional responses to pain.[20–22] Activation of the insula has been demonstrated in a variety of sensory and pain-inducing paradigms.[20,21,23–26] The insula has been suggested as a relay station for sensory information into the limbic system and is known to play an important role in regulation of autonomic responses. The thalamus has also been shown to be critically important in acute pain processing; activation of the thalamus has been shown in both animals[27] and human functional imaging pain studies.[21,28] Together, these regions are

thought to make up the "pain matrix"[29,30] (**Fig. 1**), which are of significant consequence in migraine.

ANATOMIC IMAGING IN MIGRAINE

Although standard anatomic imaging appears to be of limited diagnostic value in migraine, recent studies have suggested significant cortical thinning may occur within regions of the pain matrix. In addition, patients with migraine appear to be at higher risk for T2 hyperintense lesions, suggesting ischemic or degenerative processes may be involved. Early voxel-based morphometry studies focusing on gray matter thickness and density did not observe significant differences in cortical density in patients with migraine.[31] However, subsequent larger studies have noted significant reductions in gray matter density in cortical areas involved in pain processing[32–35] as well as an increase in gray matter density within the periaqueductal gray (PAG) in patients with visible T2 lesions.[32] Interestingly, in patients with migraine with visual aura, studies have identified thicker visual cortex,[36] presumably due to more frequent activation in these areas.

In addition to changes in gray matter density, several studies have suggested migraine is an

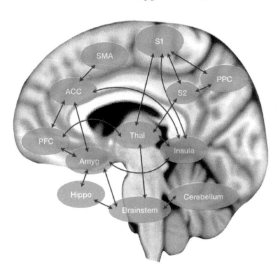

Fig. 1. The pain matrix. The pain matrix consists of the thalamus (Thal), insula, amygdala (Amyg), brainstem (including the pons and PAG), hippocampus (Hippo), prefrontal cortex (PFC), ACC, cerebellum, supplemental motor area (SMA), primary somatosensory cortex (S1), secondary somatosensory cortex (S2), and the posterior parietal cortex (PPC). (*Data from* Peyron R, Laurent B, Garcia-Larrea L. Functional imaging of brain responses to pain. A review and meta-analysis (2000). Neurophysiol Clin 2000;30:263–88; and Forss N, Raij TT, Seppa M, et al. Common cortical network for first and second pain. Neuroimage 2005;24:132–42.)

independent risk factor for deep white matter lesions.[37–40] Migraine patients appear to have an increased risk of ischemic vascular disease[41] and approximately double the risk of ischemic stroke.[42] In a cohort of 186 patients with migraine, significant associations were found between T2 hyperintense lesions and longer disease duration and higher headache frequency.[43] Prevalence of white matter T2 hyperintense lesions appears to be higher in migraine with aura compared with migraine without aura.[40] Although largely unknown, several pathologic processes have been proposed as an explanation for this higher incidence, including focal hypoperfusion, oligemia, glutamatergic excitotoxicity, immune-related demyelination, inflammation, and mitochondrial dysfunction.[39,44–46]

DIFFUSION IMAGING IN MIGRAINE

Diffusion MR changes have also been observed in patients with migraine. In particular, studies have shown higher apparent diffusion coefficient (ADC), or mean diffusivity (MD), and lower fractional anisotropy (FA) in the frontal lobe[47] along with the genu, splenium, and body of the corpus callosum,[48] consistent with microstructural alterations along these pathways. In migraine patients with aura, a reduced FA along the thalamocortical tract and reduced FA along the ventral trigeminothalamic tract have been observed,[49] whereas a reduced FA in the ventrolateral PAG has been observed in migraine patients without aura.[49] In addition, diffusion MR has revealed enhanced connectivity between temporal pole and entorhinal cortex[50] as well as high connectivity between frontal lobe regions with reduced FA and regions within the pain network (orbitofrontal cortex, insula, thalamus, and dorsal midbrain/pons).[47] Interestingly, a lower ADC has been observed in migraine patients with T2 hyperintense lesions,[51] and transient diffusion changes in the thalamus (increased FA and lower MD) have been observed during migraine without aura, which were normalized after attack.[52] Together, these observations suggest dynamic changes in water mobility may occur during the various stages of attacks.

PERFUSION AND VASCULAR IMAGING IN MIGRAINE

Most notably, CBF in patients with migraine appears significantly impaired, although the temporal changes in CBF before, during, and after migraine appear complex (Table 1). Cortical spreading depression (CSD)[53] is thought to underlie migraine visual aura,[54,55] and the early depolarization or activation phase of CSD has been shown to be associated with a transient change in CBF[54,55] and blood oxygenation.[56,57] This transient increase in CBF appears to be in conflict with work by Olesen and colleagues,[58,59] using SPECT to show focal reduction in CBF in migraine attacks with an aura. Subsequent dynamic susceptibility contrast perfusion MR imaging studies have confirmed the characteristic hypoperfusion (lower CBF) and collapsed vasculature (low cerebral blood volume with increased mean transit time) that occurs during aura in patients with migraine.[60–62] Dynamic contrast-enhanced (DCE) perfusion MR imaging, which can provide additional information about the blood-brain barrier (BBB), has similarly shown an increased CBF without increased BBB disruption in the pons/brainstem in patients with migraine.[63] These results are consistent with arterial spin labeling (ASL)[64] and perfusion studies using SPECT demonstrating similarly decreased CBF in patients with migraine.[65,66]

This reduced CBF during the onset of prolonged migraine with aura is contrasted with a substantial *increase* in CBF during the late stages of migraine[67] (see Table 1). Using ASL, lower CBF has been observed in brain regions consistent with symptoms in childhood migraine within 14 hours of aura, and higher CBF was observed after 14 hours from symptoms.[68] Similarly, ASL studies have well-documented hyperperfusion during migraine headaches after aura has occurred, but during symptom presentation.[69] DCE perfusion MR imaging case reports have suggested possible hemispheric increase in vascular permeability in migraine with aura[70] and increased CBF in the visual cortex and posterior white matter regions in migraineurs with visual aura.[63] These studies support the hypothesis that migraine with aura results in a transient, early decrease in CBF during aura formation, and a characteristic increase in CBF occurs during the late stages of migraine.

In migraine without aura, CBF changes appear less consistent across studies (see Table 1). Many studies have shown no changes in hemodynamics in migraine patients without aura,[60,71–73] whereas other studies have shown *reduced* CBF during migraine attack without aura[74,75] or significantly *higher* CBF values during the acute headache attack in the brainstem[76] or the dorsal pons.[77,78] Underscoring this inconsistency may be the spatial heterogeneity of CBF changes during migraine. For example, a study by Arkink and colleagues[79] observed complex changes in CBF throughout the brain, including an increase in CBF during attack of the inferior and middle temporal gyrus in migraine without aura, while also observing a decrease in CBF within the inferior

Table 1
Summary of brain perfusion studies in migraine headaches

Authors	Technique	Headache	Participants (N)	Conclusion	References
Gutschalk et al, 2002	DWI, MR perfusion, PET	Hemiplegic migraine	1	DWI and MR perfusion: normal; PET: reduced relative tracer uptake	Gutschalk A, et al. Neurosci Lett 2002;332:115–8.
Hsu et al, 2008	MR perfusion	Hemiplegic migraine	11	Hyperperfusion	Hsu DA, et al. Brain Dev 2008;30:86–90.
Masuzaki et al, 2001	MR perfusion	Hemiplegic migraine	1	Hyperperfusion	Masuzaki M, et al. AJNR Am J Neuroradiol 2001;22:1795–7.
Jacob et al, 2006	MR perfusion	Hemiplegic migraine	1	Hyperperfusion	Jacob A, et al. Cephalalgia 2006;26:1004–9.
Oberndorfer et al, 2004	MR perfusion	Hemiplegic migraine	1	Hyperperfusion	Oberndorfer S, Cephalalgia 2004;24:533–9.
Lindahl et al, 2002	MR perfusion	Hemiplegic migraine	1	Hyperperfusion, DWI normal	Lindahl AJ, et al. J Neurol Neurosurg Psychiatry 2002;73:202–3.
Yilmaz et al, 2009	MR perfusion, DWI	Hemiplegic migraine	1	Hypoperfusion, DWI normal	Yilmaz A, et al. Cephalalgia 2009;30:615–9.
Kraus et al, 2007	MR perfusion, DWI	Hemiplegic migraine	2	Hypoperfusion, DWI normal	Kraus J, et al. Nervenarzt 2007;78:1420–4.
Altinok et al, 2010	MR perfusion, DWI	Hemiplegic migraine	1	Hypoperfusion, small area of restricted diffusion	Altinok D, et al. Pediatr Radiol 2010;40:1958–61.
Gonzalez-Alegre, 2003	MRA	Hemiplegic migraine	1	MRA normal	Gonzalez-Alegre P & Tippin J. Headache 2003;43:72–5.
De Sanctis et al, 2011	MRA, DWI	Hemiplegic migraine	2	MRA, DWI were normal	De Sanctis S, et al. Headache 2011;51:447–50.
Barbour et al, 2001	MR imaging and MRA	Hemiplegic migraine	1	Normal	Barbour PJ. Headache 2001;41:310–6.
Kumar et al, 2009	MR imaging, DWI	Hemiplegic migraine	1	DWI normal	Kumar G, et al. Headache 2009;49:139–42.
Friberg et al, 1987	SPECT	Hemiplegic migraine	3	Hypoperfusion, preceded by focal hyperperfusion	Friberg L, et al. Brain 1987;110:917–34.
Cheng et al, 2010	SPECT	Hemiplegic migraine	30	During aura: hypoperfusion; during headache: hyperperfusion	Cheng MF, et al. Clin Nucl Med 2010;35:456–8.

frontal gyrus in migraine without aura. Taken together, current literature suggests less pronounced and more complex changes in CBF may occur in migraine patients without aura.

Some studies have suggested a possible link between vascular anomalies within the circle of Willis and decreased CBF during migraine with aura.[80] Although early MR angiography studies appeared to show no difference in incompleteness of the circle of Willis in migraine patients compared with healthy controls,[81] subsequent studies have shown a higher than expected prevalence of incomplete circle of Willis in patients with migraine.[82,83] In particular, migraine patients experiencing aura appear to have a higher prevalence of an incomplete circle of Willis,[84] whereas no elevated incidence in migraine without aura has been observed.[84,85]

FUNCTIONAL IMAGING IN MIGRAINE

The most crucial observation in functional neuroimaging in migraine has been that brainstem areas are active during pain and that after successful treatment this activation persists, whereas it is not present between attacks[76–78,86,87] (Table 2). Activated areas in the brainstem include the dorsal midbrain and dorsolateral pons, and hypothalamic activation has been described as well.[87] Increased activation of dorsolateral pons is also observed in chronic migraine,[88] and dorsal midbrain activation is consistent with reports of migrainelike headaches following stimulation in patients with implanted electrodes for chronic pain control[89,90] as well as reports of patients with lesions in these areas producing migraine symptoms.[91,92]

Task-based functional MR imaging (fMR imaging) as a clinical tool for assessing migraine is relatively limited due to the spontaneous, transient nature of these attacks and the imaging need for a planned experimental paradigm. Therefore, most functional studies in migraine have induced migraines to image the resulting changes (see Table 2). Functional tasks performed during $H_2^{15}O$-labeled PET showed increased activation in the dorsal pons,[76,86,87] midbrain,[87] brainstem, hypothalamus,[87] periaqueductal gray,[93,94] midbrain trigeminal area, and visual cortex[87] during painful stimulation. An increase in blood oxygen level–dependent (BOLD) fMR imaging signal has been observed in the extrastriate cortex and occipital cortex during induction of migraine with visual aura,[57] and increased BOLD signal in temporal pole and entorhinal cortex has been observed in both ictal and interictal migraine periods.[50] fMR imaging during visual, olfactory, or vestibular stimuli results in

greater BOLD response and hyperexcitability in visual cortex and visual network,[95–98] limbic structures,[99] and mediodorsal thalamus,[100] respectively. In addition, increased BOLD signal in ACC,[101,102] prefrontal cortex or middle frontal gyrus,[102,103] brainstem and medulla,[102] and hypothalamus[104,105] has also been observed, consistent with an increase in activation in areas involved in pain processing during invoked migraine.[106]

Functional connectivity measures using MR imaging at rest are less consistent and appear more complex, with some regions demonstrating increased connectivity and other areas demonstrating reduced connectivity as a result of migraine. For example, decreased functional connectivity within the pain-processing networks,[107] the default mode network (DMN),[108] and frontoparietal regions of the executive network (middle frontal gyrus and dorsal ACC)[109,110] have been observed. In addition, increased connectivity between PAG, hypothalamus, and/or amygdala and other brain areas within nociceptive and somatosensory processing pathways have also been detected.[111–114]

METABOLIC AND MOLECULAR IMAGING IN MIGRAINE

In addition to functional alterations, patients with migraine also appear to have altered brain metabolism and biochemistry (Table 3). PET with ^{18}F-fluorodeoxyglucose (FDG) studies have demonstrated increased activation of the vestibulothalamocortical pathway and decreased metabolism in the visual cortex during spontaneous migraine attacks.[115] At rest, significant *hypometabolism* has been observed in regions involved in pain processing,[116] including bilateral insula, bilateral ACC and posterior parietal cortex, premotor, PFC, and primary somatosensory cortex. These results suggest migraine may be intimately linked with primary metabolic dysfunction as well as potential secondary effects of brain regions involved in pain processing due to repetitive headache attacks.

MR spectroscopy (MRS), a noninvasive method of investigating the biochemical composition of the brain and inferring metabolic information, has been used to highlight various biological changes within the brain in patients with migraine. Phosphorous (^{31}P)-MRS studies have implied abnormal energy metabolism, and potential mitochondrial dysfunction may occur in patients with migraine. Multiple studies have observed decreased phosphocreatine (PCr),[117–123] suggesting mitochondrial abnormalities and impaired cerebral

Table 2
Summary of brain functional imaging studies in migraine

Authors	Technique	Headache	Participants (N)	Conclusion	References
Kim et al, 2010	^{18}FDG-PET	Migraine	40	Hypometabolism in regions known to be involved in central pain processing (bilateral insula, bilateral ACC and PCC, left premotor and PFP, and left primary SSC)	Kim JH, Kim S, Suh SI, et al. Interictal metabolic changes in episodic migraine: a voxel-based FDG-PET study. Cephalalgia 2010;30(1):53–61.
Shin et al, 2014	^{18}FDG-PET	Spontaneous migraine	2	Activation of the vestibulothalamocortical pathway and decreased metabolism in the VC	Shin JH, Kim YK, Kim HJ, et al. Altered brain metabolism in vestibular migraine: comparison of interictal and ictal findings. Cephalalgia 2014;34(1):58–67.
Kassab et al, 2009	^{18}FDG-PET	Migraine	25	Metabolic disturbance in posterior white matter of cerebrum and cerebellum in migraineurs	Kassab M, Bakhtar O, Wack D, et al. Resting brain glucose uptake in headache-free migraineurs. Headaches 2009;49(1):90–7.
Hadjikhani et al, 2001	Event-related fMR imaging	Migraine with aura	3	Focal increase in BOLD signal within extrastriate cortex progressing contiguously and slowly over occipital cortex during visual aura	Hadjikhani N, Sanchez del Rio M, Wu O, et al. Mechanisms of migraine aura revealed by functional MRI in human visual cortex. Proc Natl Acad Sci U S A 2001;98(8):4687–92.
Moulton et al, 2008	Event-related fMR imaging	Migraine	24	Hypofunction of nucleus cuneiforms in migraine patients	Moulton EA, Burstein R, Tully S, et al. Interictal dysfunction of a brainstem descending modulatory center in migraine patients. PLoS One 2008;3:e3799.
Moulton et al, 2011	Event-related fMR imaging	Migraine	17	Increase BOLD response to trigeminal painful stimulation in TP and EC in migraine patients, during the interictal period	Moulton EA, Becerra L, Maleki N, et al. Painful heat reveals hyperexcitability of the temporal pole in interictal and ictal migraine states. Cereb Cortex 2011;21:435–48.
Russo et al, 2012	Event-related fMR imaging	Migraine without aura	32	Increasing BOLD response in perigenual part of ACC at 51° C, and divergent response in pons in migraine patients	Russo A, Tessitore A, Esposito F, et al. Pain processing in patients with migraine: an event-related fMRI study during trigeminal nociceptive stimulation. J Neurol 2012;259:1903–12.

Study	Imaging type	Migraine type	N	Findings	Reference
Stankewitz, 2011	Event-related fMR imaging	Migraine	40	Increased BOLD response in PFC, ACC, red nucleus, and ventral medulla in migraine patients and a decrease in HC, without changes in pain perception	Stankewitz A, May A. Increased limbic and brainstem activity during migraine attacks following olfactory stimulation. Neurology 2011;77(5):476–82.
Schulte et al, 2017	Event-related fMR imaging	Migraine	54	Significantly stronger activation of the anterior right hypothalamus in chronic migraine patients compared with HC	Schulte LH, Allers A, May A. Hypothalamus as a mediator of chronic migraine evidence from high-resolution fMRI. Neurology 2017;88(21):2011–6.
Russo et al, 2017	Event-related fMR imaging	Migraine without aura	60	Increased BOLD response in the MFG	Russo A, Esposito F, Conte F, et al. Functional interictal changes of pain processing in migraine with ictal cutaneous allodynia. Cephalalgia 2017;37(4):305–14.
Schwedt et al, 2014	Event-related fMR imaging	Migraine without aura	51	Greater activation in cortical and subcortical areas involved in pain processing in migraine patients within the interictal period	Schwedt TJ, Chong CD, Chiang CC, et al. Enhanced pain-induced activity of pain-processing regions in a case-control study of episodic migraine. Cephalalgia 2014;34(12):947–58.
Schulte et al, 2016	Event-related fMR imaging	Migraine without aura	1	Hypothalamic activity increases toward the next migraine attack; altered functional coupling between the hypothalamus, spinal trigeminal nuclei, and the dorsal rostral pons	Schulte LH, May A. The migraine generator revisited: continuous scanning of the migraine cycle over 30 days and three spontaneous attacks. Brain 2016;139(Pt 7):1987–93.
Martin et al, 2011	Event-related fMR imaging	Migraine	38	Hyperexcitability of the VC with a wider photoresponsive area in migraine patients during interictal periods	Martin H, Sanchez del Rio M, de Silanes CL, et al. Photoreactivity of the occipital cortex measured by functional magnetic resonance imaging-blood oxygenation level dependant in migraine patients and healthy volunteers: pathophysiological implications. Headache 2011;51(10):1520–8.
Datta et al, 2013	Event-related fMR imaging	Migraine	75	Greater response to visual stimulation within primary VC and lateral geniculate nuclei in patients with migraine without aura compared with patients with migraine without aura and HC	Datta R, Aguirre GK, Hu S, et al. Interictal cortical hyperresponsiveness in migraine is directly related to the presence of aura. Cephalalgia 2013;33:365–74.

(continued on next page)

Table 2
(continued)

Authors	Technique	Headache	Participants (N)	Conclusion	References
Hougaard et al, 2014	Event-related fMR imaging	Migraine with aura	20	Greater response in cortical area, which belongs to an advanced visual network (ie, inferior parietal and frontal gyrus, superior parietal lobule)	Hougaard A, Amin FM, Hoffman MB, et al. Interhemispheric differences of fMRI responses to visual stimuli in patients with side-fixed migraine aura. Hum Brain Mapp 2014;35(6):2714–23.
Stankewitz et al, 2010	Event-related fMR imaging	Migraine	20	Greater BOLD response in limbic structures as well as in the RoP in migraine patients during spontaneous and untreated attacks	Stankewitz A, Voit HL, Bingel U, et al. A new trigemino-nociceptive stimulation model for event-related fMRI. Cephalalgia 2010;30:475–85.
Russo et al, 2014	Event-related fMR imaging	Migraine without aura	24	Greater response to vestibular stimuli in mediodorsal thalamus in patients with VM relative to both patients with migraine without aura and HC	Russo A, Marcelli V, Esposito F, et al. Abnormal thalamic function in patients with vestibular migraine. Neurology 2014;82(23):2120–6.
Weiller et al, 1995	$H_2{}^{15}O$-labeled PET	Spontaneous migraine	9	Activation in brainstem DoP, persistent even after injection of sumatriptan	Weiller C, May A, Limmroth V, et al. Brainstem activation in spontaneous human migraine attacks. Nat Med 1995;1(7):658–60.
Afridi et al, 2005	$H_2{}^{15}O$-labeled PET	Induced migraine	6	Activation in DoP during migraine attack, ipsilateral to side of pain, in migraine patients	Afridi SK, Giffin NJ, Kaube H, et al. A positron emission tomographic study in spontaneous migraine. Arch Neurol 2005;62(8):1270–5.
Denuelle et al, 2007	$H_2{}^{15}O$-labeled PET	Migraine	7	Activations in midbrain, pons, and hypothalamus during migraine attack and headache relief by sumatriptan	Denuelle M, Fabre N, Payoux P, et al. Hypothalamic activation in spontaneous migraine attacks. Headache 2007;47(10):1418–26.
Denuelle et al, 2007	$H_2{}^{15}O$-labeled PET	Migraine	7	Activation in VC by luminous stimulation during migraine attack and after headache relief but not during interictal period	Denuelle M, Fabre N, Payoux P, et al. Hypothalamic activation in spontaneous migraine attacks. Headache 2007;47(10):1418–26.

Study	Imaging modality	Group	N	Findings	Reference
Maniyar et al, 2014	H_2 ^{15}O-labeled PET	Induced migraine	8	Activations in the posterolateral hypothalamus, midbrain tegmental area, PAG, DP, and various cortical areas	Maniyar FH, Sprenger T, Monteith T, et al. Brain activations in the premonitory phase of nitroglycerin-triggered migraine attacks. Brain 2014;137(Pt 1):232–41.
Maniyar et al, 2014	H_2 ^{15}O-labeled PET	Induced migraine	27	Activation in brain circuits mediating nausea such rostral dorsal medulla and PAG	Maniyar FH, Sprenger T, Schankin C, et al. The origin of nausea in migraine—a PET study. J Headache Pain 2014;15:84.
Boulloche et al, 2010	H_2 ^{15}O-labeled PET	Migraine	14	VC hyperexcitability potentiated by the concomitant heat pain stimulation	Boulloche N, Denuelle M, Payoux P, et al. Photophobia in migraine: an interictal PET study of cortical hyperexcitability and its modulation by pain. J Neurol Neurosurg Psychiatry 2010;81(9):978–84.
Denuelle et al, 2008	H_2 ^{15}O-labeled PET	Migraine	7	Activations in midbrain, pons, and hypothalamus during migraine attack and headache relief by sumatriptan	Denuelle M, Fabre N, Payoux P, et al. Posterior cerebral hypoperfusion in migraine without aura. Cephalalgia 2008;28(8):856–62.
Denuelle et al, 2011	H_2 ^{15}O-labeled PET	Migraine	8	Activation in visual cortex by luminous stimulation during migraine attack and after headache relief but not during interictal period	Denuelle M, Boulloche N, Payoux P, et al. A PET study of photophobia during spontaneous migraine attacks. Neurology 2011;76(3):213–8.
Dermarquay et al, 2008	H_2 ^{15}O-labeled PET	Migraine	23	Activation in piriform cortex and anterosuperior temporal gyrus in olfactory hypersensitivity and odor-triggered headache attack in migraineurs	Demarquay G, Royet JP, Mick G, et al. Olfactory hypersensitivity in migraineurs: a H(2) (15)O-PET study. Cephalalgia 2008;28(10):1069–80.
Coppola et al, 2017	Resting-state fMR imaging	Migraine	32	Increased FC between MPFC and both PCC and bilateral insula	Coppola G, Di Renzo A, Tinelli E, et al. Resting state connectivity between default mode network and insula and encodes acute migraine headache. Cephalalgia 2017;1:3331024177152230.
Mainero et al, 2010	Resting-state fMR imaging	Migraine	34	Decrease functional resting-state connectivity between PAG and brain regions involved in pain processing	Mainero C, Boshyan J, Hadjikhani N. Altered functional magnetic resonance imaging resting-state connectivity in periaqueductal gray networks in migraine. Ann Neurol 2011;70(5):838–45.

(continued on next page)

Table 2
(continued)

Authors	Technique	Headache	Participants (N)	Conclusion	References
Tessitore et al, 2013	Resting-state fMR imaging	Migraine	40	Decreased FC in prefrontal and temporal regions of DMN in migraine patients	Tessitore A, Russo A, Giordano A, et al. Disrupted default mode network connectivity in migraine without aura. J Headache Pain 2013;14:89.
Russo et al, 2012	Resting-state fMR imaging	Migraine without aura	28	Reduction in the MFG and the ACC in migraine patients with migraine without aura	Russo A, Tessitore A, Giordano A, et al. Executive resting-state network connectivity in migraine without aura. Cephalalgia 2012;32(14):1041–8.
Tessitore et al, 2015	Resting-state fMR imaging	Migraine with aura	60	Reduction in the MFG and the ACC in migraine patients with migraine with aura	Tessitore A, Russo A, Conte F, et al. Abnormal connectivity within executive resting-state network in migraine with aura. Headache 2015;55(6):794–805.
Tedeschi et al, 2016	Resting-state fMR imaging	Migraine with aura	60	Significant increased FC in the right lingual gyrus within the RS visual in patients with migraine with aura	Tedeschi G, Russo A, Conte F, et al. Increased interictal visual network connectivity in patients with migraine with aura. Cephalalgia 2016;36(2):139–47.
Niddam et al, 2015	Resting-state fMR imaging	Migraine with aura	78	Reduced FC between salience and visual networks in patients with migraine with aura	Niddam DM, Lai KL, Fuh JL, et al. Reduced functional connectivity between salience and visual networks in migraine with aura. Cephalalgia 2015;36(1):53–66.
Hougaard et al, 2015	Resting-state fMR imaging	Migraine with aura	80	No abnormalities of intrinsic brain connectivity in the interictal phase of migraine with aura	Hougaard A, Amin FM, Magon S, et al. No abnormalities of intrinsic brain connectivity in the interictal phase of migraine with aura. Eur J Neurol 2015;22(4):702–e46.

Study	Imaging	Population	N	Findings	Reference
Zhao et al, 2013	Resting-state fMR imaging	Migraine without aura	60	Neuronal dysfunction in the thalamus, brainstem, and temporal pole in patients with long-term disease duration compared with patients with short-term disease duration and HC	Zhao L, Liu J, Dong X, et al. Alterations in regional homogeneity assessed by fMRI in patients with migraine without aura stratified by disease duration. J Headache Pain 2013;14:85.
Moulton et al, 2014	Resting-state fMR imaging	Migraine without aura	24	Increased FC between the hypothalamus and brain areas that regulate sympathetic and parasympathetic functions	Moulton EA, Becerra L, Johnson A, et al. Altered hypothalamic functional connectivity with autonomic circuits and the locus coeruleus in migraine. PLoS One 2014;9(4):e95508.
Hadjikhani et al, 2013	Resting-state fMR imaging	Migraine	82	Increased FC between the amygdala and visceroceptive insula in migraine patients	Hadjikhani N, Ward N, Boshyan J, et al. The missing link: enhanced functional connectivity between amygdala and visceroceptive cortex in migraine. Cephalalgia 2013;33(15):1264–8.
Yu et al, 2012	Resting-state fMR imaging	Migraine without aura	52	Decreased ReHo values in supplementary motor area, rostral anterior cingulate, prefrontal and orbitofrontal cortices in migraineurs	Yu D, Yuan K, Zhao L, et al. Regional homogeneity abnormalities in patients with interictal migraine without aura: a resting-state study. NMR Biomed 2012;25(5):806–12.
Cao et al, 1999	Task-related fMR imaging	Migraine	18	Activation of the red nucleus and substantia nigra in association with visually triggered symptoms of migraine	Cao Y, Welch KM, Aurora S, et al. Functional MRI-BOLD of visually triggered headache in patients with migraine. Arch Neurol 1999;56(5):548–54.
Antal et al, 2011	Task-related fMR imaging	Migraine	36	Hyperresponsivness of the VC beyond visual areas in migrainous even in the interictal period	Antal A, Polania R, Saller K, et al. Differential activation of the middle-temporal complex to visual stimulation in migraineurs. Cephalalgia 2011;31(3):338–45.

(continued on next page)

Table 2
(continued)

Authors	Technique	Headache	Participants (N)	Conclusion	References
Vincent et al, 2003	Task-related fMR imaging	Migraine with aura	10	Activation in extrastriate visual cortex contralaterally to the side of stimulation in migraineurs	Vincent M, Pedra E, Mourao-Miranda J, et al. Enhanced interictal responsiveness of the migraineous visual cortex to incongruent activation bar stimulation: a functional MRI visual activation study. Cephalalgia 2003;23(9): 860–8.
Bramanti et al, 2005	Task-related fMR imaging	Migraine with aura	1	Different activation patterns in occipital cortex during headache attack and interictal	Bramanti P, Grugno R, Vitetta A, et al. Ictal and interictal hypoactivation of the occipital cortex in migraine with aura. A neuroimaging and electrophysiological study. Funct Neurol 2005;20(4):169–71.
Huang et al, 2006	Task-related fMR imaging	Migraine with aura	20	No differences in visual cortical activation in migraineurs compared with HC	Huang J, DeLano M, Cao Y. Visual cortical inhibitory function in migraine is not generally impaired: evidence from a combined psychophysical test with an fMRI study. Cephalalgia 2006;26(5):554–60.
Stankewitz et al, 2011	Task-related fMR imaging	Migraine	40	Lower activations in trigeminal nuclei during interictal; increased activation in dorsal pons	Stankewitz A, Aderjan D, Eippert F, et al. Trigeminal nociceptive transmission in migraineurs predicts migraine attacks. J Neurosci 2011;31(6):1937–43.

Table 3
Summary of brain molecular and metabolic imaging in migraine

Authors	Technique	Headache	Participants (N)	Conclusion	References
Aguila et al, 2015	¹H-MRS	Migraine	38	GABA + increased in MX vs controls; suggest altered excitability of cortical neurons during the interictal period. GABA + included detection of nonspecified macromolecules, which might cause contamination of the results	Aguila M-ER, et al. NMR Biomed 2015;28:890–7.
Arngrim et al, 2016	¹H-MRS	Migraine	29	No differences in MA during hypoxia-induced headaches vs controls; suggest no mitochondrial dysfunction	Arngrim N, et al. Brain 2106;139:723–737.
Becerra et al, 2016	¹H-MRS	Migraine	65	No differences in MO + MA vs controls; post hoc analysis: cross-validation test using quadratic discriminant analysis model showed that glutamine, NAA, and aspartate as a group differentiate MO + MA from control; suggest a "complex" of metabolite alterations, which may underlie changes in neuronal chemistry in the migraine brain, supporting the theory of the hyperexcitable migraine brain	Becerra L, et al. Neuroimage Clin 2016;11:588–94.
Bigal et al, 2008	¹H-MRS	Migraine	28	GABA decreased in MO + MA with severe migraine attacks in the month before MRS vs controls; suggest that it may indicate reduced inhibition	Bigal ME, et al. Neurology 2008;70:2078–80.
Bridge et al, 2015	¹H-MRS	Migraine	26	GABA ~10% decreased in MA vs controls; suggest reduced inhibition occipitally in MA consistent with occipital hyperexcitability. Positive correlation between glutamate and BOLD activation in the visual cortex during visual stimulation in MA vs controls Suggests enhanced glutamate activation; altogether, the results suggest an abnormal excitation-inhibition coupling in the occipital cortex. The MA cohort reported visual stimuli as a migraine trigger	Bridge H, et al. Cephalalgia 2015;35:1025–30.
Dichgans et al, 2005	¹H-MRS	Migraine	32	Differences measured in cerebellum for FHM1 vs controls; suggest neuronal impairment (NAA), altered glial cell proliferation (myoinositol) and impaired glutamatergic neurotransmission	Dichgans M, et al. Neurology 2005;64:608–13.

(continued on next page)

Table 3
(continued)

Authors	Technique	Headache	Participants (N)	Conclusion	References
Fayed et al, 2014	¹H-MRS	Migraine	216	No differences in MX vs controls	Fayed N, et al. Acad Radiol 2014;21:1211–7.
Gonzales de la Aleja et al, 2013	¹H-MRS	Migraine	46	Glutamate increased in MA + MO vs controls in the anterior paracingulate cortex; suggests altered excitability and increased susceptibility to migraine triggers. Glutamate/glutamine ratio abnormal in MO + MA vs controls in the occipital cortex; suggests abnormal neuronal-glial coupling of glutamatergic metabolism or increased neuron/astrocyte ratio in the occipital cortex	Gonzales de la Aleja J, et al. Headache 2013;53:365–75.
Grimaldi et al, 2010	¹H-MRS	Migraine	14	No differences in FHM2 vs controls	Grimaldi D, et al. Cephalalgia 2010;30:522–59.
Gu et al, 2008	¹H-MRS	Migraine	34	NAA/choline decreased in left thalamus in MO vs controls; suggest mitochondrial and neuronal dysfunction due to neuronal deafferentation in the thalamus	Gu T, et al. Neurol Res 2008;30:229–33.
Lai et al, 2011	¹H-MRS	Migraine	88	NAA increased in EM in pons bilaterally compared with CM and controls; no differences between CM vs controls; suggest neuronal hypertrophy at the dorsal pons in EM. 23/53 CM patients were diagnosed with MOH	Lai T, et al. J Headache Pain 2011;12:295–302.
Lirng et al, 2015	¹H-MRS	Migraine	30	Myo-inositol increased in MX with depression vs MX without depression; no healthy controls; suggest glial dysfunction in dorsolateral prefrontal cortex in migraineurs with depression	Lirng J, et al. Cephalagia 2015;35:702–9.
Macri et al, 2003	¹H-MRS	Migraine	15	Choline decreased in MA vs controls; suggest membrane composition alterations. Only study to report choline alterations	Macri M, et al. J Magn Reson Imaging 2003;21:1201–6.
Mohamed et al, 2013	¹H-MRS	Migraine	32	NAA decreased in MO vs controls; NAA more decreased in right thalamus vs left thalamus in MO. NAA decreased, lactate and myoinositol increased with increased duration and attack frequency in MO; suggest altered energy metabolism correlated to severity of disease	Mohamed RE, et al. Egypt J Radiol Nucl Med 2013;44:859–70.

Study	Technique	Condition	N	Findings	Reference
Prescot et al, 2009	¹H-MRS	Migraine	18	No differences in MX vs controls; linear discriminant analysis showed a separation between MX and controls based on NAAG and glutamine in ACC and insula; suggest glutamatergic abnormalities in ACC and insula	Prescot A, et al. Mol Pain 2009;5:34.
Reyngoudt et al, 2011	¹H-MRS	Migraine	40	No differences in MO vs controls before or after visual stimulation; argue against a significant switch to nonaerobic glucose metabolism during long-lasting photic stimulation of the visual cortex in MO	Reyngoudt H, et al. J Headache Pain 2011;12:295–302.
Sandor et al, 2005	¹H-MRS	Migraine	21	Lactate increased in MA with visual aura vs FHM/SHM and vs controls before, during, and after visual stimulation in visual cortices; suggest mitochondrial dysfunction	Sandor P, et al. Cephalalgia 2005;25:507–18.
Sarchielli et al, 2005	¹H-MRS	Migraine	54	NAA decreased at baseline and after visual stimulation in MA vs MO and vs controls; no differences in MO vs controls; suggest less efficient mitochondrial function in MA	Sarichielli P, et al. Neuroimage 2005;24:1025–31.
Schulz et al, 2007	¹H-MRS	Migraine	37	No difference between MA and SHM + FHM vs controls; lactate peaks undetectable	Schulz UG, et al. Brain 2007;130:3102–10.
Siniatchkin et al, 2012	¹H-MRS	Migraine	20	Glutamine + Glutamate (Glx) increased at baseline in MA vs controls; suggests excessive glutamate mediated excitation in migraine. Both anodal and cathodal transcranial direct current stimulation caused Glx decrease in MA, which did not increase to baseline after visual stimulation as in controls; suggest abnormal cortical information processing and excitability in migraineurs mediated by altered glutamatergic neurotransmission	Siniatchkin M, et al. Cereb Cortex 2012;22:2207–16.
Wang et al, 2006	¹H-MRS	Migraine	37	No differences in CM vs controls suggest that the hypothalamus might not play a pivotal role in chronic migraine	Wang S, et al. J Neurol Neurosurg Psychiatry 2006;77:622–5.
Watanabe et al, 1996	¹H-MRS	Migraine	12	Lactate increased in a small heterogeneous group of patients: migraine with visual aura (N = 3), basilar type migraine (N = 1), and migrainous infarction (N = 2) vs controls (N = 6); suggest mitochondrial dysfunction. The participants had last attack within 2 mo before testing	Watanabe H, et al. Neurology 1996;47:1093–5.

(continued on next page)

Table 3
(continued)

Authors	Technique	Headache	Participants (N)	Conclusion	References
Zielman et al, 2014	¹H-MRS	Migraine	37	NAA decreased in SHM + FHM1 + FHM2 vs controls in cerebellum; NAA more decreased in FHM1 vs controls than SHM and FHM2; suggest neuronal loss or dysfunction in the cerebellum and/or less efficient mitochondrial function. Glx and myo-inositol not measured in pons	Zielman R, et al. Cephalalgia 2014;34:959–67.
Barbiroli et al, 1990	³¹P-MRS	Migraine	23	PCr decreased in MpA + MS vs controls; suggest mitochondrial abnormalities as a potential cause to defects in oxidative metabolism, making cells not meet energy demand	Barbiroli B, Montagna P, Cortelli P, et al. Complicated migraine studied by phosphorus magnetic resonance spectroscopy. Cephalalgia 1990;10:263–72.
Barbiroli et al, 1992	³¹P-MRS	Migraine	24	Significant changes in MA vs controls; only ³¹P-MRS study to report decreased pHi; indicates increased lactate levels. Collectively, the data suggest less freely available energy in the cell and abnormal oxidative metabolism due to mitochondrial dysfunction	Barbiroli B, et al. Neurology 1992;42:1209–14.
Boska et al, 2002	³¹P-MRS	Migraine	86	Magnesium decreased in FHM + SHM vs controls in the posterior region, including the occipital lobe; suggested to contribute to the cortical hyperexcitability. PDE increased in MO vs controls in the posterior region including the occipital lobe; suggested that this might be a compensatory mechanism to maintain membrane stability. Data not shown for ADP	Boska MD, et al. Neurology 2002;58;1227–33.
Lodi et al, 1997	³¹P-MRS	Migraine	27	Significant changes in MA vs controls. Collectively, these data suggest impaired cerebral oxidative metabolism and abnormal mitochondrial function, unable to meet increased energy demand. Only ³¹P-MRS study to report increased pHi; indicates decreased lactate levels; suggested to be due to ionic abnormalities in the brain causing dysfunction of proton pumps. The cohorts were juvenile	Lodi R, et al. Pediatr Res 1997;42:866–71.

Lodi et al, 2001	^{31}P-MRS	Migraine	107	Magnesium and $\Delta G_{ATP\ hyd}$ decreased in all groups vs controls. The data suggest reduced release of free energy by ATP hydrolysis due to mitochondrial dysfunction, thus magnesium levels are downregulated to reequilibrate the rapidly available free energy. $\Delta G_{ATP\ hyd}$ is defined as the freely available energy released by ATP hydrolysis in the intact cell, calculated based on ATP, ADP, Pi, and magnesium. Data not shown for PCr, Pi, and ADP	Lodi R, et al. Brain Res Bull 2001;54:437–41.
Montagna et al, 1994	^{31}P-MRS	Migraine	40	Significant changes in MO vs controls. Collectively, the data suggest a defect and altered energy metabolism.	Montagna P, et al. Neurology 1994;44:666–9.
Ramadan et al, 1989	^{31}P-MRS	Migraine	44	Magnesium decreased ictally in MO pMg (N = 10) vs controls; suggest that low magnesium promotes CSD, thus initiating the migraine attack. No patient was tested both ictally and interictally; none had aura during testing. Data not shown for PCr, Pi, ADP, and ATP	Ramadan NM, et al. Headache 1989;29:590–3.
Reyngoudt et al, 2010	^{31}P-MRS	Migraine	44	PCr, PP, and ATP decreased in MO vs controls. Collectively, the data suggest an impaired energy metabolism, and the decreased ATP level further suggests presence of a mitochondrial component in migraine. ATP was more decreased in a subgroup with the highest attack frequency. Only ^{31}P-MRS study to determine the absolute (ATP) and not calculate other metabolite concentrations based on assumed (ATP) = 3.0 mmol/L	Reyngoudt H, et al. Cephalalgia 2010;31:1243–53.
Schulz et al, 2007	^{31}P-MRS	Migraine	37	Cr/Pi decreased and Pi/ATP increased in sporadic and familiar hemiplegic migraine (N = 9) vs migraine with nonmotor aura (N = 10) in gray matter; suggest alterations in the energy metabolism	Schulz UG, et al. Brain 2007;130:3102–10.
Uncini et al, 1995	^{31}P-MRS	Migraine	35	Significant changes in family members (N = 5) vs controls suggest abnormal energy metabolism due to mitochondrial dysfunction. Differences reported for 5 family members, whereof 2 have no history of migraine, vs controls	Unicini A, et al. J Neurol Sci 1995;129:214–22.

(continued on next page)

Table 3
(continued)

Authors	Technique	Headache	Participants (N)	Conclusion	References
Welch et al, 1988	^{31}P-MRS	Migraine	47	No differences in pHi ictally (N = 11) or interictally (N = 9) in MO + MA vs controls; indicates no lactate alteration. Data not shown for ADP and ATP. Data for PCr and Pi are reported in Welch et al[37] No ictal vs interictal state comparison; no patient had aura during testing, and the results were compared with controls who were not age- and gender-matched	Welch KMA, et al. Cephalalgia 1988;8:273–7.
Welch et al, 1989	^{31}P-MRS	Migraine	47	PCr decreased and Pi increased ictally (N = 11) in MO pMA vs controls. Pi increased interictally (N = 9) in MO pMA vs controls; suggest an altered energy metabolism during migraine attacks. No difference in pHi; suggests no lactate alteration. Data not shown for ADP and ATP. No ictal vs interictal state comparison. No patient had aura during testing, and the results were compared with controls who were not age and gender matched	Welch KMA, et al. Neurology 1989;39:538–41.
Wall et al, 2005	PET and [carbonyl-11C] zolmitriptan	Migraine	8	Rapid dose-proportional uptake of ^{11}C-zolmitriptan into the brain	Wall A, Kågedal M, Bergstrom M, et al. Distribution of zolmitriptan into the CNS in healthy volunteers: a positron emission tomography study. Drugs RD 2005;6(3):139–47.
Da Silva et al, 2014	PET with 11C-carfentanil	Spontaneous migraine	12	μOR activation in the ictal phase in the medial PFC, strongly associated with the μOR availability level during the interictal phase	Da Silva AF, Nascimento TD, DosSantos MF, et al. Association of micro-opioid activation in the prefrontal cortex with spontaneous migraine attacks—brief report I. Ann Clin Transl Neurol 2014;1(6):439–44

Da Silva et al, 2014	PET with 11C-carfentanil	Spontaneous migraine	1	Reduction in μOR in the pain-modulatory regions of the endogenous micro-opioid system during the migraine attack	Da Silva AF, Nascimento TD, Love T, et al. 3D-neuronavigation in vivo through a patient's brain during a spontaneous migraine headache. J Vis Exp 2014;(88).
Chabriat et al, 1995	PET with 18F-fluorosetoperone	Migraine	12	No differences of cortical 5-HT2 receptors' distribution volumes in migraine patients when compared with HC	Chabriat H, Tehindrazanarivelo A, Vera P, et al. 5HT2 receptors in cerebral cortex of migraineurs studied using PET and 18F-fluorosetoperone. Cephalalgia 1995;15(2):104–8.
Demarquay et al, 2011	PET with a 5-HT1A radioligand	Migraine	20	Increased 5-HT1A receptors in the pontine raphe during odor-triggered migraine attack	Demarquay G, Lothe A, Royet JP, et al. Brainstem changes in 5-HT1A receptor availability during migraine attack. Cephalalgia 2011;3(1):84–94.
Chugani et al, 1999	PET with alpha-[11C] methyl-L-tryptophan tracer	Migraine without aura	19	Increased rate of brain 5-HT synthesis in the ictal phase of migraine attack	Chugani DC, Niimura K, Chaturvedi S, et al. Increased brain serotonin synthesis in migraine. Neurology 1999;53(7):1473–9.

oxidative metabolism as potential causes of migraine. Using proton (^{1}H)-MRS, reports have shown altered excitability of the brain in patients with migraine, including abnormal levels of neurotransmitters glutamate and γ-aminobutyrate acid (GABA) in the occipital cortex, cingulate cortex, and other areas implicated in pain processing.[124–129] In addition, lower levels of N-acetyl aspartate (NAA), a neuronal marker, was observed in migraineurs with aura who had T2 hyperintense lesions[51] within the occipital lobe[128,130] as well as the thalamus[131] and cerebellum.[132]

In addition, serotonergic function and serotonin (5-HT) receptors have been implicated in migraine pathogenesis,[133] leading to several PET studies examining 5-HT being performed.[134] PET imaging using ^{18}F-fluorosetoperone (a 5-HT2-specific radioligand), however, did not show any differences in the distribution of 5-HT2 receptors in the cortex.[135] A study using an α-[^{11}C]methyl-L-tryptophan tracer did show an increased rate of brain 5-HT synthesis during the acute phase of migraine attacks,[136] which was subsequently verified using a specific antagonist of 5-HT receptors,[137] suggesting that increased 5-HT1A receptor availability is present during migraine attacks, particularly within the pontine raphe.[135,138]

SUMMARY

In summary, the use of advanced imaging in routine diagnostic practice appears to provide only limited value in adult and pediatric patients with migraine who have not experienced changes in headache quality or associated symptoms. However, advanced imaging may have potential for studying the biological manifestations and pathophysiology of migraine headaches. Migraine with aura appears to have characteristic spatiotemporal changes in structural anatomy, function, hemodynamics, metabolism, and biochemistry, whereas migraine without aura appears more complex. Large, controlled, multicenter imaging-based observational trials are needed to confirm the abundant anecdotal evidence in the literature and test the variety of scientific hypotheses thought to underscore migraine pathophysiology.

REFERENCES

1. Medina LS, D'Souza B, Vasconcellos E. Adults and children with headache: evidence-based diagnostic evaluation. Neuroimaging Clin N Am 2003; 13:225–35.
2. Evans RW. Diagnostic testing for the evaluation of headaches. Neurol Clin 1996;14:1–26.
3. Jordan JE. Expert panel on neurologic, I. Headache. AJNR Am J Neuroradiol 2007;28:1824–6.
4. Goadsby PJ, Lipton RB, Ferrari MD. Migraine—current understanding and treatment. N Engl J Med 2002;346:257–70.
5. Global Burden of Disease Study 2013 Collaborators. Global, regional, and national incidence, prevalence, and years lived with disability for 301 acute and chronic diseases and injuries in 188 countries, 1990-2013: a systematic analysis for the Global Burden of Disease Study 2013. Lancet 2015;386: 743–800.
6. Lance JW. Current concepts of migraine pathogenesis. Neurology 1993;43:S11–5.
7. Stewart WF, Ricci JA, Chee E, et al. Lost productive time and cost due to common pain conditions in the US workforce. JAMA 2003;290:2443–54.
8. Andlin-Sobocki P, Jonsson B, Wittchen HU, et al. J. Cost of disorders of the brain in Europe. Eur J Neurol 2005;12(Suppl 1):1–27.
9. May A. A review of diagnostic and functional imaging in headache. J Headache Pain 2006;7:174–84.
10. Demaerel P, Boelaert I, Wilms G, et al. The role of cranial computed tomography in the diagnostic work-up of headache. Headache 1996;36:347–8.
11. Sotaniemi KA, Rantala M, Pyhtinen J, et al. Clinical and CT correlates in the diagnosis of intracranial tumours. J Neurol Neurosurg Psychiatry 1991;54: 645–7.
12. Wang HZ, Simonson TM, Greco WR, et al. Brain MR imaging in the evaluation of chronic headache in patients without other neurologic symptoms. Acad Radiol 2001;8:405–8.
13. Detsky ME, McDonald DR, Baerlocher MO, et al. Does this patient with headache have a migraine or need neuroimaging? JAMA 2006; 296:1274–83.
14. Sempere AP, Porta-Etessam J, Medrano V, et al. Neuroimaging in the evaluation of patients with non-acute headache. Cephalalgia 2005;25:30–5.
15. Silberstein SD. Practice parameter: evidence-based guidelines for migraine headache (an evidence-based review): report of the Quality Standards Subcommittee of the American Academy of Neurology. Neurology 2000;55:754–62.
16. Edlow JA, Panagos PD, Godwin SA, et al. Clinical policy: critical issues in the evaluation and management of adult patients presenting to the emergency department with acute headache. Ann Emerg Med 2008;52:407–36.
17. Becker WJ, Findlay T, Moga C, et al. Guideline for primary care management of headache in adults. Can Fam Physician 2015;61:670–9.
18. Sandrini G, Friberg L, Jänig W, et al. Neurophysiological tests and neuroimaging procedures in non-acute headache: guidelines and recommendations. Eur J Neurol 2004;11:217–24.

19. May A, Kaube H, Büchel C, et al. Experimental cranial pain elicited by capsaicin: a PET study. Pain 1998;74:61–6.

20. Hsieh JC, Hannerz J, Ingvar M. Right-lateralised central processing for pain of nitroglycerin-induced cluster headache. Pain 1996;67:59–68.

21. Casey KL, Minoshima S, Berger KL, et al. Positron emission tomographic analysis of cerebral structures activated specifically by repetitive noxious heat stimuli. J Neurophysiol 1994;71:802–7.

22. Jones AK, Friston K, Frackowiak RS. Localization of responses to pain in human cerebral cortex. Science 1992;255:215–6.

23. Coghill RC, Talbot JD, Evans AC, et al. Distributed processing of pain and vibration by the human brain. J Neurosci 1994;14:4095–108.

24. Hsieh JC, Ståhle-Bäckdahl M, Hägermark O, et al. Traumatic nociceptive pain activates the hypothalamus and the periaqueductal gray: a positron emission tomography study. Pain 1996;64:303–14.

25. Burton H, Videen TO, Raichle ME. Tactile-vibration-activated foci in insular and parietal-opercular cortex studied with positron emission tomography: mapping the second somatosensory area in humans. Somatosens Mot Res 1993;10:297–308.

26. Derbyshire SW, Jones AK, Devani P, et al. Cerebral responses to pain in patients with atypical facial pain measured by positron emission tomography. J Neurol Neurosurg Psychiatry 1994;57:1166–72.

27. Goadsby PJ, Zagami AS, Lambert GA. Neural processing of craniovascular pain: a synthesis of the central structures involved in migraine. Headache 1991;31:365–71.

28. Rosen SD, Paulesu E, Frith CD, et al. Central nervous pathways mediating angina pectoris. Lancet 1994;344:147–50.

29. Peyron R, Laurent B, Garcia-Larrea L. Functional imaging of brain responses to pain. A review and meta-analysis (2000). Neurophysiol Clin 2000;30: 263–88.

30. Forss N, Raij TT, Seppa M, et al. Common cortical network for first and second pain. Neuroimage 2005;24:132–42.

31. Matharu MS, Good CD, May A, et al. No change in the structure of the brain in migraine: a voxel-based morphometric study. Eur J Neurol 2003;10: 53–7.

32. Rocca MA, Ceccarelli A, Falini A, et al. Brain gray matter changes in migraine patients with T2-visible lesions: a 3-T MRI study. Stroke 2006;37: 1765–70.

33. Valfre W, Rainero I, Bergui M, et al. Voxel-based morphometry reveals gray matter abnormalities in migraine. Headache 2008;48:109–17.

34. Kim JH, Suh SI, Seol HY, et al. Regional grey matter changes in patients with migraine: a voxel-based morphometry study. Cephalalgia 2008;28:598–604.

35. Yu ZB, Peng J, Lv YB, et al. Different mean thickness implicates involvement of the cortex in migraine. Medicine (Baltimore) 2016;95:e4824.

36. Gaist D, Hougaard A, Garde E, et al. Migraine with visual aura associated with thicker visual cortex. Brain 2018. https://doi.org/10.1093/brain/awx382.

37. Kruit MC, van Buchem MA, Hofman PA, et al. Migraine as a risk factor for subclinical brain lesions. JAMA 2004;291:427–34.

38. Kruit MC, Launer LJ, Ferrari MD, et al. Infarcts in the posterior circulation territory in migraine. The population-based MRI CAMERA study. Brain 2005;128:2068–77.

39. Kruit MC, Launer LJ, Ferrari MD, et al. Brain stem and cerebellar hyperintense lesions in migraine. Stroke 2006;37:1109–12.

40. Kruit MC, van Buchem MA, Launer LJ, et al. Migraine is associated with an increased risk of deep white matter lesions, subclinical posterior circulation infarcts and brain iron accumulation: the population-based MRI CAMERA study. Cephalalgia 2010;30:129–36.

41. Bigal ME, Kurth T, Hu H, et al. Migraine and cardiovascular disease: possible mechanisms of interaction. Neurology 2009;72:1864–71.

42. Kurth T, Chabriat H, Bousser MG. Migraine and stroke: a complex association with clinical implications. Lancet Neurol 2012;11:92–100.

43. Trauninger A, Leél-Ossy E, Kamson DO, et al. Risk factors of migraine-related brain white matter hyperintensities: an investigation of 186 patients. J Headache Pain 2011;12:97–103.

44. Dodick DW, Roarke MC. Crossed cerebellar diaschisis during migraine with prolonged aura: a possible mechanism for cerebellar infarctions. Cephalalgia 2008;28:83–6.

45. Longoni M, Ferrarese C. Inflammation and excitotoxicity: role in migraine pathogenesis. Neurol Sci 2006;27(Suppl 2):S107–10.

46. Sparaco M, Feleppa M, Lipton RB, et al. Mitochondrial dysfunction and migraine: evidence and hypotheses. Cephalalgia 2006;26:361–72.

47. Szabo N, Kincses ZT, Párdutz A, et al. White matter microstructural alterations in migraine: a diffusion-weighted MRI study. Pain 2012;153: 651–6.

48. Li XL, Fang YN, Gao QC, et al. A diffusion tensor magnetic resonance imaging study of corpus callosum from adult patients with migraine complicated with depressive/anxious disorder. Headache 2011; 51:237–45.

49. DaSilva AF, Granziera C, Tuch DS, et al. Interictal alterations of the trigeminal somatosensory pathway and periaqueductal gray matter in migraine. Neuroreport 2007;18:301–5.

50. Moulton EA, Becerra L, Maleki N, et al. Painful heat reveals hyperexcitability of the temporal pole

in interictal and ictal migraine States. Cereb Cortex 2011;21:435–48.

51. Aradi M, Schwarcz A, Perlaki G, et al. Quantitative MRI studies of chronic brain white matter hyperintensities in migraine patients. Headache 2013;53: 752–63.

52. Coppola G, Tinelli E, Lepre C, et al. Dynamic changes in thalamic microstructure of migraine without aura patients: a diffusion tensor magnetic resonance imaging study. Eur J Neurol 2014;21: 287-e213.

53. Leao AAP. Spreading depression of activity in the cerebral cortex. J Neurophysiol 1944;7:359–90.

54. Lauritzen M. Regional cerebral blood flow during cortical spreading depression in rat brain: increased reactive hyperperfusion in low-flow states. Acta Neurol Scand 1987;75:1–8.

55. Mraovitch S, Calando Y, Goadsby PJ, et al. Subcortical cerebral blood flow and metabolic changes elicited by cortical spreading depression in rat. Cephalalgia 1992;12:137–41 [discussion: 127].

56. Cao Y, Welch KM, Aurora S, et al. Functional MRI-BOLD of visually triggered headache in patients with migraine. Arch Neurol 1999;56:548–54.

57. Hadjikhani N, Sanchez Del Rio M, Wu O, et al. Mechanisms of migraine aura revealed by functional MRI in human visual cortex. Proc Natl Acad Sci U S A 2001;98:4687–92.

58. Olesen J, Larsen B, Lauritzen M. Focal hyperemia followed by spreading oligemia and impaired activation of rCBF in classic migraine. Ann Neurol 1981;9:344–52.

59. Friberg L, Olesen J, Lassen NA, et al. Cerebral oxygen extraction, oxygen consumption, and regional cerebral blood flow during the aura phase of migraine. Stroke 1994;25:974–9.

60. Sanchez del Rio M, Bakker D, Wu O, et al. Perfusion weighted imaging during migraine: spontaneous visual aura and headache. Cephalalgia 1999;19:701–7.

61. Blicher JU, Tietze A, Donahue MJ, et al. Perfusion and pH MRI in familial hemiplegic migraine with prolonged aura. Cephalalgia 2016;36:279–83.

62. Forster A, Wenz H, Kerl HU, et al. Perfusion patterns in migraine with aura. Cephalalgia 2014;34: 870–6.

63. Hougaard A, Amin FM, Christensen CE, et al. Increased brainstem perfusion, but no blood-brain barrier disruption, during attacks of migraine with aura. Brain 2017;140:1633–42.

64. Kato Y, Araki N, Matsuda H, et al. Arterial spin-labeled MRI study of migraine attacks treated with rizatriptan. J Headache Pain 2010;11:255–8.

65. Oberndorfer S, Wöber C, Nasel C, et al. Familial hemiplegic migraine: follow-up findings of diffusion-weighted magnetic resonance imaging (MRI), perfusion-MRI and [99mTc] HMPAO-SPECT in a

patient with prolonged hemiplegic aura. Cephalalgia 2004;24:533–9.

66. Takase Y, Nakano M, Tatsumi C, et al. Clinical features, effectiveness of drug-based treatment, and prognosis of new daily persistent headache (NDPH): 30 cases in Japan. Cephalalgia 2004;24: 955–9.

67. Mourand I, Menjot de Champfleur N, Carra-Dallière C, et al. Perfusion-weighted MR imaging in persistent hemiplegic migraine. Neuroradiology 2012;54:255–60.

68. Boulouis G, Shotar E, Dangouloff-Ros V, et al. Magnetic resonance imaging arterial-spin-labelling perfusion alterations in childhood migraine with atypical aura: a case-control study. Dev Med Child Neurol 2016;58:965–9.

69. Pollock JM, Deibler AR, Burdette JH, et al. Migraine associated cerebral hyperperfusion with arterial spin-labeled MR imaging. AJNR Am J Neuroradiol 2008;29:1494–7.

70. Rotstein DL, Aviv RI, Murray BJ. Migraine with aura associated with unilateral cortical increase in vascular permeability. Cephalalgia 2012;32: 1216–9.

71. Olesen J, Lauritzen M, Tfelt-Hansen P, et al. Spreading cerebral oligemia in classical- and normal cerebral blood flow in common migraine. Headache 1982;22:242–8.

72. Olesen J, Friberg L, Olsen TS, et al. Timing and topography of cerebral blood flow, aura, and headache during migraine attacks. Ann Neurol 1990;28: 791–8.

73. Lauritzen M, Olesen J. Regional cerebral blood flow during migraine attacks by Xenon-133 inhalation and emission tomography. Brain 1984;107(Pt 2):447–61.

74. Friberg L, Olesen J, Iversen H, et al. Interictal "patchy" regional cerebral blood flow patterns in migraine patients. A single photon emission computerized tomographic study. Eur J Neurol 1994;1:35–43.

75. Friberg L, Olesen J, Iversen HK, et al. Migraine pain associated with middle cerebral artery dilatation: reversal by sumatriptan. Lancet 1991;338: 13–7.

76. Weiller C, May A, Limmroth V, et al. Brain stem activation in spontaneous human migraine attacks. Nat Med 1995;1:658–60.

77. Bahra A, Matharu MS, Buchel C, et al. Brainstem activation specific to migraine headache. Lancet 2001;357:1016–7.

78. Afridi SK, Matharu MS, Lee L, et al. A PET study exploring the laterality of brainstem activation in migraine using glyceryl trinitrate. Brain 2005;128: 932–9.

79. Arkink EB, Bleeker EJ, Schmitz N, et al. Cerebral perfusion changes in migraineurs: a voxelwise

comparison of interictal dynamic susceptibility contrast MRI measurements. Cephalalgia 2012; 32:279–88.

80. Cucchiara B, Detre J. Migraine and circle of Willis anomalies. Med Hypotheses 2008;70:860–5.

81. Paemeleire K, Proot P, De Keyzer K, et al. Magnetic resonance angiography of the circle of Willis in migraine patients. Clin Neurol Neurosurg 2005; 107:301–5.

82. Bugnicourt JM, Garcia PY, Peltier J, et al. Incomplete posterior circle of willis: a risk factor for migraine? Headache 2009;49:879–86.

83. Cavestro C, Richetta L, L'episcopo MR, et al. Anatomical variants of the circle of willis and brain lesions in migraineurs. Can J Neurol Sci 2011;38: 494–9.

84. Cucchiara B, Wolf RL, Nagae L, et al. Migraine with aura is associated with an incomplete circle of willis: results of a prospective observational study. PLoS One 2013;8:e71007.

85. Ezzatian-Ahar S, Amin FM, Obaid HG, et al. Migraine without aura is not associated with incomplete circle of Willis: a case-control study using high-resolution magnetic resonance angiography. J Headache Pain 2014;15:27.

86. Afridi SK, Giffin NJ, Kaube H, et al. A positron emission tomographic study in spontaneous migraine. Arch Neurol 2005;62:1270–5.

87. Denuelle M, Fabre N, Payoux P, et al. Hypothalamic activation in spontaneous migraine attacks. Headache 2007;47:1418–26.

88. Matharu MS, Bartsch T, Ward N, et al. Central neuromodulation in chronic migraine patients with suboccipital stimulators: a PET study. Brain 2004;127: 220–30.

89. Raskin NH, Hosobuchi Y, Lamb S. Headache may arise from perturbation of brain. Headache 1987; 27:416–20.

90. Veloso F, Kumar K, Toth C. Headache secondary to deep brain implantation. Headache 1998;38: 507–15.

91. Haas DC, Kent PF, Friedman DI. Headache caused by a single lesion of multiple sclerosis in the periaqueductal gray area. Headache 1993;33:452–5.

92. Goadsby PJ. Neurovascular headache and a midbrain vascular malformation: evidence for a role of the brainstem in chronic migraine. Cephalalgia 2002;22:107–11.

93. Maniyar FH, Sprenger T, Monteith T, et al. Brain activations in the premonitory phase of nitroglycerin-triggered migraine attacks. Brain 2014;137: 232–41.

94. Maniyar FH, Sprenger T, Schankin C, et al. The origin of nausea in migraine-a PET study. J Headache Pain 2014;15:84.

95. Boulloche N, Denuelle M, Payoux P, et al. Photophobia in migraine: an interictal PET study of cortical hyperexcitability and its modulation by pain. J Neurol Neurosurg Psychiatry 2010;81: 978–84.

96. Martin H, Sánchez del Río M, de Silanes CL, et al. Photoreactivity of the occipital cortex measured by functional magnetic resonance imaging-blood oxygenation level dependent in migraine patients and healthy volunteers: pathophysiological implications. Headache 2011;51:1520–8.

97. Datta R, Aguirre GK, Hu S, et al. Interictal cortical hyperresponsiveness in migraine is directly related to the presence of aura. Cephalalgia 2013;33:365–74.

98. Hougaard A, Amin FM, Hoffmann MB, et al. Interhemispheric differences of fMRI responses to visual stimuli in patients with side-fixed migraine aura. Hum Brain Mapp 2014;35:2714–23.

99. Stankewitz A, Voit HL, Bingel U, et al. A new trigemino-nociceptive stimulation model for event-related fMRI. Cephalalgia 2010;30:475–85.

100. Russo A, Marcelli V, Esposito F, et al. Abnormal thalamic function in patients with vestibular migraine. Neurology 2014;82:2120–6.

101. Russo A, Tessitore A, Esposito F, et al. Pain processing in patients with migraine: an event-related fMRI study during trigeminal nociceptive stimulation. J Neurol 2012;259:1903–12.

102. Stankewitz A, May A. Increased limbic and brainstem activity during migraine attacks following olfactory stimulation. Neurology 2011;77:476–82.

103. Russo A, Esposito F, Conte F, et al. Functional interictal changes of pain processing in migraine with ictal cutaneous allodynia. Cephalalgia 2017;37: 305–14.

104. Schulte LH, Allers A, May A. Hypothalamus as a mediator of chronic migraine: evidence from high-resolution fMRI. Neurology 2017;88:2011–6.

105. Schulte LH, May A. The migraine generator revisited: continuous scanning of the migraine cycle over 30 days and three spontaneous attacks. Brain 2016;139:1987–93.

106. Schwedt TJ, Chong CD, Chiang CC, et al. Enhanced pain-induced activity of pain-processing regions in a case-control study of episodic migraine. Cephalalgia 2014;34:947–58.

107. Colombo B, Rocca MA, Messina R, et al. Resting-state fMRI functional connectivity: a new perspective to evaluate pain modulation in migraine? Neurol Sci 2015;36(Suppl 1):41–5.

108. Tessitore A, Russo A, Giordano A, et al. Disrupted default mode network connectivity in migraine without aura. J Headache Pain 2013;14:89.

109. Russo A, Tessitore A, Giordano A, et al. Executive resting-state network connectivity in migraine without aura. Cephalalgia 2012;32:1041–8.

110. Tessitore A, Russo A, Conte F, et al. abnormal connectivity within executive resting-state network in migraine with Aura. Headache 2015;55:794–805.

111. Mainero C, Boshyan J, Hadjikhani N. Altered functional magnetic resonance imaging resting-state connectivity in periaqueductal gray networks in migraine. Ann Neurol 2011;70:838–45.

112. Zhao L, Liu J, Dong X, et al. Alterations in regional homogeneity assessed by fMRI in patients with migraine without aura stratified by disease duration. J Headache Pain 2013;14:85.

113. Moulton EA, Becerra L, Johnson A, et al. Altered hypothalamic functional connectivity with autonomic circuits and the locus coeruleus in migraine. PLoS One 2014;9:e95508.

114. Hadjikhani N, Ward N, Boshyan J, et al. The missing link: enhanced functional connectivity between amygdala and visceroceptive cortex in migraine. Cephalalgia 2013;33:1264–8.

115. Shin JH, Kim YK, Kim HJ, et al. Altered brain metabolism in vestibular migraine: comparison of interictal and ictal findings. Cephalalgia 2014;34:58–67.

116. Kim JH, Kim S, Suh SI, et al. Interictal metabolic changes in episodic migraine: a voxel-based FDG-PET study. Cephalalgia 2010;30:53–61.

117. Barbiroli B, Montagna P, Cortelli P, et al. Complicated migraine studied by phosphorus magnetic resonance spectroscopy. Cephalalgia 1990;10:263–72.

118. Barbiroli B, Montagna P, Cortelli P, et al. Abnormal brain and muscle energy metabolism shown by 31P magnetic resonance spectroscopy in patients affected by migraine with aura. Neurology 1992;42:1209–14.

119. Lodi R, Iotti S, Cortelli P, et al. Deficient energy metabolism is associated with low free magnesium in the brains of patients with migraine and cluster headache. Brain Res Bull 2001;54:437–41.

120. Montagna P, Cortelli P, Monari L, et al. 31P-magnetic resonance spectroscopy in migraine without aura. Neurology 1994;44:666–9.

121. Reyngoudt H, Paemeleire K, Descamps B, et al. 31P-MRS demonstrates a reduction in high-energy phosphates in the occipital lobe of migraine without aura patients. Cephalalgia 2011;31:1243–53.

122. Schulz UG, Blamire AM, Corkill RG, et al. Association between cortical metabolite levels and clinical manifestations of migrainous aura: an MR-spectroscopy study. Brain 2007;130:3102–10.

123. Uncini A, Lodi R, Di Muzio A, et al. Abnormal brain and muscle energy metabolism shown by 31P-MRS in familial hemiplegic migraine. J Neurol Sci 1995;129:214–22.

124. Bridge H, Stagg CJ, Near J, et al. Altered neurochemical coupling in the occipital cortex in migraine with visual aura. Cephalalgia 2015;35:1025–30.

125. Gonzalez de la Aleja J, Ramos A, Mato-Abad V, et al. Higher glutamate to glutamine ratios in occipital regions in women with migraine during the interictal state. Headache 2013;53:365–75.

126. Siniatchkin M, Sendacki M, Moeller F, et al. Abnormal changes of synaptic excitability in migraine with aura. Cereb Cortex 2012;22:2207–16.

127. Aguila ME, Lagopoulos J, Leaver AM, et al. Elevated levels of GABA+ in migraine detected using (1) H-MRS. NMR Biomed 2015;28:890–7.

128. Dichgans M, Herzog J, Freilinger T, et al. 1H-MRS alterations in the cerebellum of patients with familial hemiplegic migraine type 1. Neurology 2005;64:608–13.

129. Fayed N, Andres E, Viguera L, et al. Higher glutamate+glutamine and reduction of N-acetylaspartate in posterior cingulate according to age range in patients with cognitive impairment and/or pain. Acad Radiol 2014;21:1211–7.

130. Sarchielli P, Tarducci R, Presciutti O, et al. Functional 1H-MRS findings in migraine patients with and without aura assessed interictally. Neuroimage 2005;24:1025–31.

131. Gu T, Ma XX, Xu YH, et al. Metabolite concentration ratios in thalami of patients with migraine and trigeminal neuralgia measured with 1H-MRS. Neurol Res 2008;30:229–33.

132. Zielman R, Teeuwisse WM, Bakels F, et al. Biochemical changes in the brain of hemiplegic migraine patients measured with 7 tesla 1H-MRS. Cephalalgia 2014;34:959–67.

133. Hamel E. Serotonin and migraine: biology and clinical implications. Cephalalgia 2007;27:1293–300.

134. Aurora SK, Barrodale PM, Tipton RL, et al. Brainstem dysfunction in chronic migraine as evidenced by neurophysiological and positron emission tomography studies. Headache 2007;47:996–1003 [discussion: 1004–7].

135. Chabriat H, Tehindrazanarivelo A, Vera P, et al. 5HT2 receptors in cerebral cortex of migraineurs studied using PET and 18F-fluorosetoperone. Cephalalgia 1995;15:104–8 [discussion: 177].

136. Chugani DC, Niimura K, Chaturvedi S, et al. Increased brain serotonin synthesis in migraine. Neurology 1999;53:1473–9.

137. Demarquay G, Lothe A, Royet JP, et al. Brainstem changes in 5-HT1A receptor availability during migraine attack. Cephalalgia 2011;31:84–94.

138. Russo A, Tessitore A, Giordano A, et al. The pain in migraine beyond the pain of migraine. Neurol Sci 2012;33(Suppl 1):S103–6.

Moving?

Make sure your subscription moves with you!

To notify us of your new address, find your **Clinics Account Number** (located on your mailing label above your name), and contact customer service at:

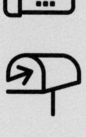

Email: journalscustomerservice-usa@elsevier.com

800-654-2452 (subscribers in the U.S. & Canada)
314-447-8871 (subscribers outside of the U.S. & Canada)

Fax number: 314-447-8029

Elsevier Health Sciences Division
Subscription Customer Service
3251 Riverport Lane
Maryland Heights, MO 63043

*To ensure uninterrupted delivery of your subscription, please notify us at least 4 weeks in advance of move.

Printed and bound by CPI Group (UK) Ltd, Croydon, CR0 4YY

03/10/2024

01040308-0014